19.95

The Alcoholism Problems:
Selected Issues

Sidney Cohen has degrees in Pharmacy and Medicine, and was awarded a Doctor of Sciences degree from Columbia University in 1976.

Dr. Cohen has researched LSD for the past 20 years and marihuana for the past 5. He has published over 250 articles and 5 books in the areas of psychopharmacology and drug abuse. He is editor of the *Drug Abuse & Alcoholism Newsletter* and is on the editorial board of *Psychosomatics*, the *International Journal of Addictions*, *Drug Dependence*, the *American Journal of Drug and Alcohol Abuse*, the *Journal of Psychoactive Drugs*, and *Substance and Alcohol Misuse*.

Dr. Cohen served as Director of the Division of Narcotic Addiction and Drug Abuse, NIMH, from 1968 to 1970. He is now a Clinical Professor of Psychiatry at Neuropsychiatric Institute, UCLA. He consults in substance abuse matters for the National Institute on Drug Abuse, the Food and Drug Administration, and the Department of the Army. He has spoken on all aspects of the drug problem in the United States and abroad.

The Alcoholism Problems: Selected Issues

Sidney Cohen, M.D.

 The Haworth Press, New York

The Haworth Press, Inc., 28 East 22 Street, New York, New York 10010

Earlier versions of chapters 1, 7, 8, 9, 11, 12, 13, 14, 23, 24, and 25 in this book were published in the Vista Hill Foundation's *Drug Abuse & Alcoholism Newsletter*, volumes 1–11, 1972–1982. Earlier versions of chapters 2, 3, 4, 5, 6, 10, 15, 16, 17, 18, 19, 20, 21, 22, 26, 27, 28, 29, 30, and 31 were published in both *Drug Abuse & Alcoholism Newsletter* and in *The Substance Abuse Problems* by Sidney Cohen, New York: The Haworth Press, Inc., 1981.

Cover design by Sonia Rabin

Library of Congress Cataloging in Publication Data

Cohen, Sidney, 1939–
    The alcoholism problems.

    Includes bibliographical references and index.
    1. Alcoholism—Addresses, essays, lectures.
I.   Title.
HV5035.C63 1983   616.86'1   83–179
ISBN 0–86656–209–5
ISBN 0–86656–179–X (pbk.)

Printed in the United States of America

CONTENTS

72119

FOREWORD

There are many books on alcohol and alcoholism. What we really need is a volume that is responsive to some of the current issues, one that provides a clarification of certain puzzling aspects of this sometimes destructive, but socially acceptable, beverage. Any book that deals with, or at least raises, some of the questions that are listed here is a worthy effort.

1. Why do we hold such diverse opinions about ethyl alcohol—opinions that range from its being an *eau vital* to the proposition that it is a protoplasmic poison?

2. Is alcoholism a weakness of character, a disease, a learned maladaptive behavior, or a response to life stress? All of the above? None of the above?

3. How strongly does advertising and the media influence our drinking behaviors?

4. How should social policy be changed? Should we: Increase taxes? Control outlets? Raise the drinking age? Regulate hours of access?

5. How do we best educate the young about dealing with this pleasant, but sometimes disastrous, beverage?

6. Does the latter-day hedonism that seems to prevail—a mind-set that has as its first commandment: "Thou shalt feel no pain"—mean that a further surge of chemical euphoria is upon us?

Yes, the personal and social causations are evident, but what about the pharmacologic imperatives that ethanol exerts? Have the rewards (and the rewarding punishments) of intoxication and befuddlement been underestimated?

Sidney Cohen is exceedingly well qualified to deal with these and other formidable questions. It is not only his long list of clinical/scientific honors. It is the nature of the man, himself. Teacher, writer, researcher, advisor, clinician, but above all, perennial student. These are his background qualifications. And, readily apparent to those who know him, he is an objective, fair, and knowledgeable participant/observer of the national and international substance-abuse scene.

His information is sound, and—uniquely these days—he actually thinks about the data. As you will see, his writing style is lucid. He challenges the reader to reflect on the strange and ambiguous relationship we have with this colorless, pungent fluid whose negative impact is almost beyond all calculation.

Jokichi Takamine, M.D.
Alcohol Research Center
Neuropsychiatric Institute
Los Angeles, California

PREFACE

The current issues and controversies about beverage alcohol and its potential disorders have been selected for consideration in this volume. Not all of the short essays are problem oriented. Some were written because new and pertinent knowledge has recently come forth.

The love-hate affair we have with this potable fluid is remarkable and complex. It is our only socially approved euphoriant, despite the fact that it becomes a dysphoriant in larger doses. Many use it to treat their mood disorders, but after a while, anxiety and depression are often increased. Perhaps this is one of the many reasons for its compulsive use. We tend to forget the unpleasant intervals and remember the feelings of relaxation and good cheer. After it increases our level of tension and unhappiness, we naturally reach for the bottle.

If all the alcohol-induced deaths were counted together, the total would compete with cancer and heart disease for the number one spot on the mortality lists, since many cancer and cardiac deaths are alcohol related. And yet this society retains a benign image of the intoxicant.

The dichotomies about alcohol will remain. We must try to understand them and must shape policies that will decrease the noxious effects of this drug while retaining its benefits.

It is a pleasure to thank the Vista Hill Foundation for their permission to reprint these articles, which first appeared in their *Drug Abuse & Alcoholism Newsletter*.

The Alcoholism Problems:
Selected Issues

I

THE NATURE
OF ALCOHOL

1. The Blood Alcohol Concentration

The blood alcohol concentration (BAC) or blood alcohol level (BAL) is a reliable and reproducible measurement of ethanol in the blood. Since alcohol diffuses uniformly to all tissues, it is also a reflection of brain ethanol levels. Breath alcohol determinations are more frequently used for practical purposes and are converted by a factor of about 2,300 so that the apparatus automatically provides a BAC reading. Breath alcohol determinations should not be done within 15 minutes of the ingestion of a drink; otherwise false elevations will occur in some cases because of the retention of ingested alcohol in the oropharynx. Urine alcohol tests only generally reflect the BAC and are not worth performing for practical purposes.

BAC READINGS

Three different ways of reporting the BAC are used, and this may lead to occasional confusion. Examples of each are given below for the BAC that is legally assumed to be an intoxicating level.

	G/100 ml	mg/100 ml	G/liter
	or	or	or
		mg/dl	
		or	
	%	mg/%	promille
	0.1 =	100 =	1.0

In this chapter, percent is used. It is converted to mg % by multiplying by 1,000. Promille is used in a number of other countries.

THE BAC AND DRIVING

The legal limit for intoxication throughout most of the United States is 0.1 percent. In some states this amount is presumptive evidence of intoxication; in others it is *per se* evidence, meaning that a finding of 0.1 percent or above in itself proves intoxication. Supporting evidence is unnecessary for conviction. Most European countries have lowered their level to 0.08 percent or lower. The World Health Organization recommends a 0.05 percent limit. A number of investigators have found that driving skills start becoming impaired at 0.04 percent. By the time a BAC of 0.1 percent is reached the probability of auto accidents rises to seven or eight times the level for sober drivers.

The BAC determines the punishment for driving-while-intoxicated arrests in a country like Denmark. For BACs between 0.08 and 0.12 percent, the fine is automatically a month's salary after taxes. From 0.121 to 0.15 percent, it is a month's salary plus loss of one's driver's license for one year. When the BAC is found to be 0.151 or higher, the offender is imprisoned for 10 days and loses his license for two years. Thus, the BAC is relied upon to mete out punishment. This is one of the few instances where a biological test is used to determine the severity of a sentence.

THE BAC AND DRINKING

Although the BAC is quite reliable, the variance is ±10 percent. Therefore, two tests are preferable to a single determination. The test is not a measure of the amount of ethanol consumed. The weight of the person is very important; likewise, the rapidity of drinking, the time elapsed since the last drink, the particular ability of the drinker to metabolize alcohol, the presence of food in the gastrointestinal tract, and other factors will determine the BAC. For example, a person weighing 100 pounds will have a BAC of about 0.22 after consuming five drinks within an hour. A 200 pound individual will have a BAC approximating 0.11 percent under the same circumstances.

A standard drink is defined as either 12 ounces of beer, 5 ounces of dry wine, or 1.5 ounces of 80 proof liquor. These quantities contain approximately the same amount of alcohol. Alcoholic beverages between 4 and 44 percent provide similar BACs. Below that percentage the alcohol absorption may be delayed by the large fluid volume. Above that percentage pylorospasm may delay absorption. The notion that whiskey produces drunkenness quicker than the more dilute beverages is probably due to the greater rapidity of its ingestion.

About 90 percent of the alcohol consumed is metabolized by liver-produced enzymes, particularly alcohol dehydrogenase. The rate of oxidation is fairly uniform for each person, averaging 0.015 percent of the BAC per hour with a range of 0.012 to 0.018 percent. This is equivalent to the metabolism of 1 gram of pure alcohol for every 10 kg of body weight per hour.

The rate of destruction of alcohol is independent of the BAC except at levels above 0.3 percent, when other enzymes like catalase and the microsomal endoplasmic oxidizing system of the liver come into play. The remaining 10 percent of the ingested alcohol is excreted unchanged by the lungs and kidneys with small amounts eliminated by the skin. It is difficult to accelerate the metabolism of alcohol, but physical exercise can increase it somewhat. The mechanism may be increased via breath and sweat excretion.

Although intestinal fermentation produces up to an ounce of ethanol a day, the alcohol dehydrogenase system is efficient enough to degrade it immediately. Therefore, a person who has taken no alcohol in beverage, medicinal, or food forms will have a BAC of 0 percent.

Since the rate of removal of alcohol from the blood is fairly constant, it is unnecessary to obtain a breath or blood sample immediately following an accident. If 4 hours have elapsed since an accident and if an estimate of the BAC at that time is desired, a sample can be taken then. To the reading that is obtained, 0.06 percent should be added (0.015 percent times 4 hours). The corrected figure will approximate the BAC at the time of the accident. Similarly, if a person goes to sleep with a BAC of 0.15 and sleeps 10 hours, he should awaken with a reading of 0 percent.

One possible error in such calculations will occur if considerable amounts of alcohol remain in the gastrointestinal tract at the time the BAC is tested. Acetaldehyde and acetate continue to be absorbed from the stomach and small intestine as ethanol is metabolically broken down. This increases the BAC, and the increase cannot be predicted. To avoid such error, BAC samples should not be obtained until 20 minutes have elapsed since the last drink.

CLINICAL CORRELATES OF THE BAC

It has been claimed that some excessive drinkers have difficulties with alcohol because they are unable to self-monitor their BAC. The importance of this factor in drinking more than was planned is not known. Training patients who have occasional problems with overdrinking to discriminate their BACs has been attempted. They are given periodic feedback while drinking by being told what their blood alcohol level is. Patients are given training in identifying the behavioral effects that typically accompany various BACs. They are required to discontinue their consumption at some specific upper level (typically 0.065 percent). Although some success with this method has been achieved, it is far from being a proven therapy, and should not be used with chronic alcoholics.

Even given the variability of the BAC according to the factors already mentioned, it is possible to indicate some approximate clinical effects with increasing BACs. At 0.03 percent (one drink) most people will feel little or nothing. A few might note flushing and be somewhat more talkative than usual. At 0.05 percent (two drinks) some relaxation and lowering of inhibitions are observable in non-tolerant drinkers. If four or five drinks are taken within an hour, the BAC wil be about 0.1 percent. Most people will feel intoxicated at this level; others will deny intoxication, but will do poorly on psychomotor testing; and a few, perhaps those with some partial tolerance, will show no evidence of ataxia, slurred speech, or mental confusion. At BACs of 0.15 to 0.3 percent (6 to 10 drinks), a staggering gait, passing out, blacking out, or irrational behavior can occur. A BAC of 0.35 has been considered to be the LD_{50} for alcohol (a lethal dose for 50 percent of the population), but this figure has been disputed as too low by others. They suggest a level of 0.4 percent—at which point the person is comatose. On the other hand, alcoholics have been known to survive a reading of 0.5 percent or more. Such BACs can be obtained by drinking a quart of whiskey in an hour. Drinkers who have achieved tolerance to alcohol manifest less effect than non-tolerant ones at every BAC.

These approximations are given for determinations done during the ascending limb of the BAC curve. During this period the mental effects are more pronounced and the mood tends to be more euphoric. On the other hand, as the BAC declines, at equivalent blood levels the mental effects are less pronounced, and less pleasant feeling tones are experienced. The explanation of this finding—and it has been consistently reported—is not evident.

Lateral nystagmus correlates quite well with the BAC. At high BAC levels nystagmus is observed on direct gaze. At lower BACs nystagmus can be elicited by fixing on an object on the lateral periphery. With precise measurement of this phenomenon, the degree of lateral fixing that produces nystagmus can provide an estimate of the BAC. Other CNS depressants can also cause lateral nystagmus.

The National Council on Alcoholism criteria for the diagnosis of alcoholism include the following.

• A BAC of 0.1 percent encountered during a routine examination is a minor sign suggestive of alcoholism.

• A BAC of 0.15 percent or more in the absence of gross intoxication is definitely indicative of marked tolerance and therefore of alcoholism.

• A BAC of 0.3 percent at any time is also one of the minor signs that contributes to a diagnosis of alcoholism.

USES OF THE BAC

Traffic Safety

The BAC is a primary instrument in a number of aspects of motor vehicle safety control. Unsafe driving such as weaving or speeding might call for a BAC test. Accidents, especially serious ones, often require blood alcohol determinations. Routine roadside surveys take a blood or breath sample to determine the alcohol usage of a random sample of auto operators.

The BAC test is an important tool in dealing with those drivers who are under the influence. It provides objective evidence that supports or refutes the arresting officer's evaluation of the car operator. A BAC, and particularly two determinations, are given considerable weight in court and during sentencing. The mere ability to do the test has doubtless served as a deterrent to some intoxicated persons who consider driving.

Self-administered breath alcohol analyzers are available for the vehicle operator so that he can check his own alcohol level before driving. A few bars also have such portable analyzers available. Some research has been done to build breath testing or cognitive tasks into the ignition system of a car that could prevent the car from starting if the test is failed.

Court Procedures

The BAC is helpful in determining the degree of impairment so that an opinion can be formed about the specific intent to commit a criminal act. Although a 0.1 percent BAC is legal evidence of intoxication, such a level would be insufficient to make a defendant incapable of premeditating, reflecting upon, or harboring malice, or of being able to form the intent to commit the crime of which he is accused. Furthermore, a plea of diminished capacity is not a valid defense when the defendant knew that drinking alcohol could produce a disturbed mental state. If involuntary intoxication can be proven—for example, drinking under duress—then the Durham Rule would hold. This rule states that the accused is not criminally responsible if the unlawful act was the product of mental disease or a mental defect.

Research

A good deal of the biobehavioral research on alcohol uses repeated BACs to correlate with the physiologic or psychologic changes that take place. The breath and blood tests are accurate enough to be used for research purposes.

Diagnosis and Treatment

Emergency rooms often use the BAC in instances of injuries. One study has reported that in fights one or both contestants have measurable blood levels 50 percent of the time. Some physicians check breath or blood levels on routine visits. The breath procedure is quickly done and inexpensive. During the treatment of an alcoholic patient, such testing is performed to provide an objective measure of recent compliance. Other physicians will not do the test because of a concern that it interferes with the patient-physician relationship. If the arrangement is set up as a part of the treatment or contract at the outset, it is usually acceptable to the patient. Methadone maintenance clinics may do the BAC routinely, at random, or when specifically indicated.

A person first seen in coma and with the odor of alcohol on his breath should have a BAC performed to rule alcohol in or out as the cause of the coma. Many other causes of coma may be masked and remain undiagnosed if the obvious cause, alcohol, is accepted. The odor of acetone in a patient in diabetic coma resembles that of alcohol on a person's breath.

Personnel Management

Some firms include BAC testing in their drug screening program of pre-employment physicals. It is sometimes done in the medical departments of corporations in order to clarify unusual on-the-job accidents or bizarre behavior. If suspension or dismissal action is contemplated, it is desirable to have objective evidence like a BAC test of intoxication during working hours.

2. Drug X: The Most Dangerous Drug on Earth

We are justifiably concerned about the effects of mind-altering drugs upon ourselves, our families, our community, and our society. We wonder whether a day will come when some drug will appear that will destroy the fabric of our social, economic, and political structure by its disintegrating effects upon the person and the community.

What would happen if a drug came into use (let's call it drug X), and it turned out to have these widespread and devastating effects? The adverse effects would be exerted not only upon the individual, but also on those around him, and upon the entire social system. They would be extensive enough to make sociologists and economists wonder whether we will be able to afford the human and financial costs of X abuse in years to come.

Drug X is here.

What have been the documented results of the drug X pandemic in this country? Only some of the proven noxious effects can be mentioned; the entire list is too long to be detailed in this space.

1. Ten million people, including increasing numbers of teenagers, are dependent upon it, and their use of it is out of control. With one person in twenty in the land a problem Xaholic, it means that 40 million people (the afflicted and their families) are directly involved with the sequellae of destructive X usage.

2. X happens to produce a lengthy intoxicated state. This means that for many hours before coma sets in or recovery occurs, judgment is impaired, controls over behavior are diminished or absent, and motor skills are reduced. As

9

a result, intoxicated people are accident prone, not only to themselves, but also to those in their vicinity. To cite only one example of their lethality, over 25,000 traffic deaths and hundreds of thousands of injuries occurred last year in connection with excessive X use.

3. Aggressiveness as a result of the impairment of the control over one's behavior has made X the most violence-producing of all drugs. Some 90 percent of all assaults, and 50 to 60 percent of all homicides take place while the aggressor was under the influence of X. In at least two studies it was also found that half of the victims had significant blood levels of X. Most homicides occur on weekends, a period when most X is consumed.

4. Police statistics across the nation consistently report that a third to a half of all arrests are related to this drug. Police, court, jail, and probation costs are enormous.

5. Half the rapes are committed while the rapist is under the influence of X.

6. In one study 67 percent of all sexually aggressive attacks against children were committed after X had been consumed by the perpetrator. X is also strongly related to the initiation of incestuous activities with minor children.

7. The suicide rate among X addicts is 6 to 20 times higher than in the general population. Even suicide attempters have high Xism rates, with figures ranging from 13 to 50 percent above non-user levels. The role of the drug itself as an agent to commit suicide should be noted. Although it is possible to cause death from the use of X alone, the more common pattern is to combine other depressant drugs with the consumption of X. The potentiating effect of X upon sedatives, depressants, and tranquilizers is well established. Potentiation also accounts for fair numbers of accidental deaths in individuals who happen to consume sublethal quantities of X plus other depressants without suicidal intention.

8. Hundreds of thousands of families are disrupted by divorce, desertion, or separation, primarily because one or both partners are Xaholics. The children of such marriages are particularly affected by the neglect, persecution, and physical attacks to which they are exposed over many years. From studies of battered children it is becoming clear that many of the parents are chronic Xaholics. The children whose family life was made chaotic by X may, themselves, take to this same drug in the search for relief from their distressing situation.

9. Industry loses five billion dollars a year and government estimates that their X-dependent employees cost a half billion dollars each year. Poor job

performance, lateness and absenteeism, illness, waste of materials, and bad decisions are only some of the causes of the losses to production and operations.
The price of general inefficiency and the loss of key, trained personnel are in-
calculable. The total cost to society is put at more than 15 billion a year.

10. Chronic Xism causes brain damage that eventually becomes irreversible. It also causes damage to the nerves, the liver, and the pancreas. It interferes
with the uptake of vitamins and other essential nutritional factors while requir-
ing more of certain nutrients for its own metabolism. Every cell of the body
is affected by these deficiencies. Resistance to infection is diminished, and death
due to pneumonia and tuberculosis is common. Fractures and other trauma are
normal hazards for the X-intoxicated person. The life span of the chronic user
is shortened by 11 years.

11. Although tension and depression may lead to problem Xism, the pro-
tracted use of this chemical produces tension and depression. Estimates vary
and statistics tend to be inaccurate because of cover-up diagnoses, but a fifth
to a quarter of admissions to psychiatric hospitals are directly or indirectly caused
by acute or chronic X ingestion.

12. The morning after a bout of X consumption many people will complain
of headache, nausea, anorexia, shakiness, and muddled thinking. This unpleasant condition appears to deter no one from going on another bout.

13. After a prolonged binge of heavy X usage a characteristic withdrawal
syndrome may be precipitated. It consists of grand mal convulsions, a toxic
psychosis with hallucinations, and difficult-to-control tremulousness and agitation. The withdrawal syndrome carries a definite mortality risk. This frightening
condition deters hardly anyone from going on another spree.

14. Despite heated debates about drug A being a stepping stone to drug B
and so on up the drug ladder, in every survey drug X usually is the first intoxicating drug used by adolescents. If we were really serious about a stepping
stone theory leading to heroin addiction, we would be concerned about the role
of drug X. But a decision of which drug leads to which drug is pointless. The
harm that comes from X is much greater than the dangers of heroin in all
respects.

Considering the harmful and disagreeable aspects of the agent it may be difficult for those not familiar with X to understand why it popularity continues
to increase each year. They may properly ask why people continue to use the
substance long after they have lost their health, their jobs, their family, their
assets, their friends, and their self-respect. An answer is not easy to come by.
First of all, even though 10 percent of the using population are in trouble with

the drug, 90 percent are not—at least, not at present. All those who use X socially have the firm conviction that they are in the 90 percent group, and most of the people in the 10 percent group think that they are also in the 90 percent group. Therefore, a major problem is the complete lack of insight into one's own condition with regards to his X habit. This permits a denial of the reality situation for a long time, often for a lifetime.

Additional factors include the "pushing" and "dealing" activities of the supplies and users, and the strong cultural acceptance of the drug. Regarding the latter point, we symbolically equate the use of X with manliness (and womanliness) and with friendliness and social enjoyment. Certain behaviors like fighting, not approved while sober, are more apt to be tolerated if the individual is intoxicated with X. The mass media portrays X-taking as a pattern of prestige, and we all laugh at the sloppy, Xonked-out character on the screen. In this country it is difficult to be an X abstainer, although there are a few of these.

A further reason for the enormous consumption of X must be mentioned. In low doses many people report feelings of relaxation, well-being, and gregariousness. In addition, some will assert that they enjoy the taste of X. It is these low-dose properties which make X attractive, and they account for its role as a social lubricant. Unfortunately, society has not found a way to prevent the transition to the social, psychological, physiological, and economic toxicity of the chronic, high-dose state.

All sorts of legal policies have proven ineffective. Prohibition of X is hardly considered these days in view of the disastrous experience with a prohibition experiment of half a century ago. It is currently freely available and openly sold. In some states only the original packages can be purchased, but in most parts of the country it can be bought by the single dose or by the car load. A meal can hardly be ordered, a plane flight taken, a conference attended (even those on Xism), to say nothing of a visit to friends without being invited to down some form of X. People have been known to feel rejected or insulted when the invitation is refused. Controls over sale extend only to minors, Indians, and Election Day closing of X stores. The situation is so grotesque that X is not even considered a drug, and a package insert is not included with each purchase.

Prevention and education efforts have, in general, been ineffective. Attempts to teach the facts about X are received with disinterest and apathy. Scare tactics about X are unnecessary, because the facts are scary as they are.

What seem to be needed is an entirely new cultural attitude toward X in which it is recognized for what it is—a dangerous drug, dangerous for 10 million people, their families, and those around them. How this new attitude can be achieved is, unfortunately, obscure.

X has to be an imaginary drug. It is inconceivable that an advanced society would put up with the tragedy of X.

BIBLIOGRAPHY

- Amir, M. Patterns in forcible rape. University of Chicago Press, Chicago, 1970.
- Bennett, R.M., *et al*. Alcohol and human physical aggression. Quart. J. Studies Alcohol. 30:870, 1969.
- Blum, R.H. Presidents Commission on Law Enforcement and Administration of Justice, Task Force Report, Washington, D.C. Government Printing Office, 1967.
- Blum, R.H. National Commission on Causes and Prevention of Violence, Staff Report. Washington, D.C. Government Printing Office, 1969.
- Goodwin, D.W. Alcohol in suicide and homicide. Quart. J. Studies Alcohol. 34:144, 1973.
- Shupe, L.M. Alcohol and crime. J. Crim. Law and Criminal. 44:661, 1964.
- Tinklenberg, J.R. Alcohol and violence, in Fox, R. and Bourne, P. (eds). Alcoholism: Progress in Research and Treatment, Academic Press, 1973.
- Wolfgang, M.E. Patterns in criminal homicide. Science Editions. New York, John Wiley and Sons, 1966.

3. Drug X: Another Point of View

This chapter was contributed by Dr. Robert A. Moore, Medical Director of the Mesa Vista Hospital, San Diego, California.

In the preceding essay Dr. Sidney Cohen refers to drug X as "the most dangerous drug on earth." Quite obviously, Dr. Cohen is referring to alcohol and the many tragic consequences of excessive alcohol use.

He presents compelling data and conclusions about the many sad consequences of alcohol use: impaired health, early death, family breakups, highway traffic fatalities, homicide, suicide, sexual assaults, and huge losses in industry from impaired productivity. Hard to measure are the harmful effects upon children raised in a family where one or both parents are alcohol abusers because it affects both their image of themselves as potential adults and their attitudes towards alcohol use for the future. Hospitals and jails find their clientele heavily represented by alcohol abusers. One certainly cannot dispute the major impact of these conclusions, and it would be foolhardy to defend alcohol abuse as a socially desirable behavior.

There is a less clearly stated point of view in the presentation: that there is an inherent risk in drinking alcohol, even in moderate or low dosage, because of the implication that everybody considers himself or herself a normal drinker, but perhaps all drinkers are vulnerable. There is a tone resembling "the myth of social drinking" presented by Dr. Max Hayman several years ago.

While Dr. Cohen recognizes attempts at legal prohibition in the past were not effective, he wonders if a new cultural attitude could be developed towards alcohol, recognizing it "for what it is—a dangerous drug." He then ends by saying "how this new attitude can be achieved is, unfortunately, obscure."

There is ample literature with quite adequate documentation outlining all the ill effects of alcohol abuse. There is much research showing the effects of alcohol on the various body systems, upon such societal institutions as marriage and the family, and such indirect lethal actions of alcohol as traffic fatalities. Still, the literature pours in. New grant applications are produced to study further the ill effects of alcohol. One wonders at the need to be constantly producing more arguments as to the evils of "John Barleycorn," as if by an orgy of "bad news" we will be able to undo this epidemic "that will destroy the fabric of our social, economic, and political structure by the disintegrating effects upon the person and his community." (Cohen) Our traditional treatment programs for alcoholics include lectures and films on the ill effects of alcohol upon the body. Perhaps there is an assumption inherent in this that the general public, as well as people suffering from the ill effects of alcohol, are unaware of this information and if we can simply convince them of the truth, the problem will be brought under control, both for the individual and for society. It appears the assumption is that alcoholics drink through ignorance of what they are doing and the harm they are producing. Having been better informed, they will mend their ways.

Similar education programs have been traditionally used in traffic safety: "If you drink, don't drive! If you drive, don't drink!" And, if you don't follow this admonition, you will be arrested and punished.

Despite this outpouring of "bad news," which has been increasing in volume in the past few years, there was a 32 percent increase in per capita absolute alcohol consumption in the United States between 1958 and 1971 (1), and it appears that there has been continued growth in consumption since then. This phenomenon is not limited to the United States since, during a roughly comparable period of time, there has been a 61 percent increase in West Germany, a 54 percent increase in Denmark, and an 83 percent increase in the Netherlands. And so it goes. About the only reassurance we find in the hope that education will reverse the trend is in France, where, during a comparable period of time, there has been a 9 percent decrease in alcohol consumption per capita, primarily a decrease in wine use (18 percent) offsetting a 20 percent increase in distilled beverage consumption during the same time.(1)

Drinking alcohol is hardly a new idea. "Alcoholic beverages were presumably discovered, rather than invented, in prehistoric times. Their origin is buried in antiquity, though the presence of wine and beer is well attested in archaeological records of the oldest civilizations and in the diets of most preliterate peoples."(2) Very early, man discovered beneficial effects from alcohol and developed a primitive system of production. "The near universality of alcoholic beverages imposes an irresistible inference: Man from earliest times appreciated the mood changing effects of these fluids, regarding them as useful and beneficient. In his attempts to appease or manipulate the divine or magical powers that he perceived as determining his fate—in his early groping for relatedness to the mystical forces of nature—man offered up to these forces something precious."(2) "Alcoholic beverages were obviously more suitable than any others for evoking these moods of release, mystification, and ecstasy that were sought as a way to communicate with and relate to powers that were invincible and beyond knowing. In particular, alcoholic beverages facilitated the rites of orgiastic communicants. Small wonder that Dionysus/Bacchus became the most popular of the gods among the Greeks and Romans.''(2)

Much could be said about the continued use of alcholic beverages in religious and social rituals, but it was also secularized into common use because of the pleasure it produced. A quantum step forward occurred in the fifteenth century with the discovery of the process of distillation, producing the ''spirit of wine'' leading us now to refer to distilled beverages as ''spirits.''

In our own country, it is worthy of note that total absolute consumption per capita of people 15 and older remained at a reasonably steady rate from 1850 to the mid 1960s, with the exception of a turn-down during the period of Prohibition. (3) If one were to comment in the late 1960s about alcohol consumption, one would have said that there has been no significant increase in alcohol use in our country, a rather surprising statement considering many alarming comments about the increasing epidemic. As indicated earlier, one cannot make that statement at this point in time since there has been now a rather precipitous upturn in alcohol consumption in the last few years. (1) Of particular concern is the increase in drinking among minors. (4) At the present time, various surveys, such as the Alcoholic Drinking Practice Survey in 1964 and 1965 and the Harris Survey in 1972–1974, showed that the majority of people 21 and older are drinkers. A 1974 Gallup Survey indicates that 68 percent of the population over 18 drink. The Harris Survey shows that 58 percent drink more than once a month, with 31 percent drinking less than .22 ounces of absolute alcohol a day, 18 percent drinking from .22 to 1.0 ounces of absolute alcohol a day, and 9 percent drinking over 1 ounce of absolute alcohol a day. (5)

Since alcohol has been used so long and everywhere, and since a high proportion of our adult population and now a high proportion of our teenage population are drinkers, isn't it time that we looked more into the question of why?

All the research—no matter how sophisticated and detailed—that delineates the evil effects of alcohol tells us very little about why alcohol is so popular. Yet, we continue to fund such research in a desperate hope that knowledge of the ill effects of alcohol will somehow conquer this problem. A physiological model has been developed by Virginia Davis to attempt to explain the phenomenon of addiction—suggesting that there may be the development of an abnormal alkaloid metabolite resulting from effects of acetaldehyde upon catecholamine metabolism and that this metabolite might have some addictive effect (6)—but otherwise we find little work directed towards the ''why.'' While there are varying rates of alcohol consumption and abuse in this country among ethnic groups, social classes, perhaps even personality types, the ubiquitousness of alcohol consumption and the large number of abusers in all groups suggest that alcohol has some overriding quality to it that crosses class lines, ethnicity, genetics, and personality development.

Thus, one is led to the conclusion that alcohol must do something very good, that it is a highly desirable compound for a majority of our population, and that understanding these good and wonderful qualities of alcohol may be much more important to us in trying to comprehend this phenomenon and develop some methods of control.

For example, it is much easier to gather data about the ill effects than the good effects. Marital disruption where alcohol plays a part is more measurable than marriage retention where alcohol has played a part. Are some marriages maintained partially through the influence of alcohol in softening disputes? It is easier to measure the number of children who are in emotional difficulty with drinking parents than it is to find the opposite. Are some parents softer figures as a result of alcohol in their relationship with their children? It is easier to measure how many rapists, exhibitionists, murderers, and assaulters committed their acts under the influence of alcohol than the opposite. Does alcohol help some individuals avoid loss of control? Suicide rates are quite high among alcoholics, but would this same group of people have an equal or higher suicide rate if alcohol was not available? In no way is this an attempt to dismiss the very serious effects of alcohol abuse, but rather it is an attempt to pose the opposite question to give a proper prspective.

We need to know what the "payoff" is in alcohol use. The greater the payoff or the greater the need for such a payoff, the greater the consumption will be. Thus, we may find that excessive use of alcohol is a result of payoffs that differ only in degree from those received by the normal and controlled drinker. It would be simplistic to say that many people drink because "it's expected" or because there is peer pressure. While this may be a factor, the fact that the drinking continues suggests that once one meets "drug X," a love affair is easily developed.

One area of study that may give us more knowledge of the "payoff" is attempting better to understand how we learn early in life to experience strong emotions. Krystal in his theoretical attempts to wed psychoanalytic and neurobiologic findings, suggests that affect intolerance may play a role in addictive disorders.(7, 8, 9) Alcohol may dampen strong affect in some and in others allow some expression by providing "dutch courage." This affect intolerance or the inability even to recognize its existence (alexithymia) may be a regression due to early infantile trauma or could be a biological error in the "affect thermostat" related to endogenous opiates. If there is a genetic factor predisposing to alcoholism, perhaps this is where it is operative.

Whatever the true state of affairs may be, the drinker experiences alcohol as a very rewarding substance that brings him or her back repeatedly even after hearing the "bad news." Alcoholics have a very difficult time explaining what alcohol does for them that is so rewarding. This is not surprising since problems of alexithymia and affect intolerance were established in the time of life before a cognitive capacity to explain them had developed.

Lastly, maybe some "good news" needs to be presented for the sake of a balanced view. The Second Special Report to the U.S. Congress on Alcohol and Health of 1974 reports on some interesting data from the Tecumseh Health Study being conducted in Tecumseh, Michigan by the University of Michigan Medical School. It appears that light drinking (four ounces of absolute alcohol a week or less) and heavy drinking do not appreciably affect the coronary heart disease rate in men aged 45-59 as measured by death by coronary or confirmed myocardial infarction. More startling, previously light and heavy drinkers who have stopped have an increase in coronary heart disease rates in the range of 3:1. Even correcting for such issues that would predispose towards coronaries as hypertension, heavy smoking, and high cholesterol, this trend remains. (8) Studies of mortality and alcohol do not show a clear effect of alcohol use. Certainly, heavy drinking is associated with higher mortality. The report summarizes: "All-in-all, the data on general mortality suggests that for amount of drinking, apparently unlike amount of smoking, there may be some kind of threshhold below which mortality is little affected. In the absence of further evidence, in fact, the classical "Anstie's limit" seems still to reflect the safe amount of drinking which has not substantially increased the risk of early death."(9) It is interesting to note that Dr. Anstie defined his "limit" in 1864, and that "limit" is one and a half ounces of absolute alcohol a day, which would be equivalent to between three and four ounces of whiskey, a pint of wine, or about a quart of beer.

In summary, Dr. Cohen has made some very important points about "drug X," points that need wide distribution and understanding. This is not in any way a rebuttal or dispute with Dr. Cohen and his facts but an attempt to present a balanced picture. Without the balanced view, we may be disappointed in our attempts to establish effective rehabilitation programs and, more importantly, modifications in drinking styles in our country generally referred to as "responsible drinking."

REFERENCES

1. Second Special Report to the U.S. Congress on Alcohol and Health. U.S. Department of Health, Education, and Welfare. June, 1974, p. 6.
2. First Special Report to the U.S. Congress on Alcohol and Health. U.S. Department of Health, Education, and Welfare. December, 1971, p. 5.
3. Ibid. p. 15.
4. Second Special Report. pp. 8-12.
5. Ibid. pp. 8-12.
6. Davis, V.E. and Walsh, M.J. Alcohol, amines and alkaloids: a possible biochemical basis for alcohol addiction. Science 167: 1005-1007, 1970.

7. Krystal, H. The genetic development of affects and affect regression. *The Annual of Psychoanalysis*, Vol. II. New York, International Universities Press, 1974.
8. Krystal, H. Affect tolerance. *The Annual of Psychoanalysis*. Vol. III. New York, International Universities Press, 1975.
9. Krystal, H. Alexithymia and psychotherapy. American Journal of Psychotherapy, 33: 17–31, 1979.
10. Second Special Report. pp. 91–96.
11. Ibid. pp. 104–121.

4. The Fetal Alcohol Syndrome: Alcohol as a Teratogen

"BEHOLD THOU SHALT CONCEIVE AND BEAR A SON: AND NOW DRINK NO WINE OR STRONG DRINK." JUDGES 13:7

In medicine, as in life, until the mind has been prepared to see something, it will pass unnoticed, as invisible as though it did not exist.

Only ten years ago the fetal alcohol syndrome (FAS) was rediscovered by Jones and Smith, and since then thousands of cases have been found. It was a rediscovery, not a discovery, because the ancients knew of a connection between alcohol intake during pregnancy and birth defects. It was also common folk knowledge that alcoholic women tended to have "small, shriveled children with an imperfect look."(1)

It was known that pregnant alcoholics miscarried more often than nondrinking women. As recently as 1968, Lemoine and his French colleagues (Quest. Med. 25:477, 1968) described 127 infants of chronic alcoholic females with "very peculiar facies, considerable retardation of growth in height and weight, and an increased frequency of malformations and psychomotor disturbances." Little attention was paid to this report.

THE SYNDROME

The FAS consists of a variable number of the following developmental defects.

20

1. Low birth weight and small size due to prenatal growth deficiencies. After birth, growth is also retarded. These children never catch up in size or weight.

2. Mental retardation with an average I.Q. in the 60s. It is now believed that the FAS is the third most common known cause of mental deficiency.

3. A variety of birth defects including, but not restricted to, microencephaly, short palpebral fissures, ptosis, epicanthal folds, maxillary hypoplasia, cleft palate, joint anomalies, anomalous genitalia, capillary hemangiomas, and altered palmar creases. As many as 50 percent of the children have some cardiac abnormality. The major heart defects include the Tetralogy of Fallot, septal defects, and patent ductus arteriosus.

ETIOLOGY

The cause of the FAS is unknown, but many of the defects can be explained on the basis of a profound effect of alcohol or its metabolite, acetaldehyde, on the fetal central nervous system during its earliest development. An abnormality of neuronal migration may be the pathological basis for much of the clinical picture.

Malnutrition secondary to chronic alcoholism does not seem to be the underlying mechanism since well-nourished pregnant women who drink also have produced FAS offspring. Furthermore, offspring of malnourished mothers tend to catch up in growth and weight after birth; FAS children do not.

The condition appears to be related to blood alcohol levels and the ability of alcohol to diffuse freely across the placental barrier. Therefore, intermittent binge drinking might produce such problems even if the total intake during pregnancy was modest. The entire period of gestation may be at risk, with the first trimester producing the malformations and the second and third trimesters inducing growth impairments.

The fetuses are very quiet *in utero*. This lack of movement may account for the undeveloped palmar creases, the frequency of breech presentations, and the joint anomalies. The decreased fetal activity might be due to the sedative effect of alcohol.

Since heavy drinkers also tend to be heavy smokers, the interaction with tobacco has made the question of causation difficult. The animal studies have demonstrated, however, that alcohol alone can be a teratogen to the fetus.

In one study 43 percent more alcoholic pregnant women produced FAS infants than a matched control group. Twelve percent of nonalcoholic women who drank moderately had children with anomalies consistent with the FAS.

It is estimated that about 4,000 to 5,000 children a year are born with varying degrees of the syndrome.

HOW MUCH ALCOHOL?

A safe level of alcohol consumption has not yet been determined. The National Institute for Alcohol Abuse and Alcoholism has suggested that no more than two mixed drinks or their equivalent in beer or wine be consumed daily during pregnancy. Other authorities recommend complete abstinence.

The risk factor appears to be great when more than six drinks are consumed daily. It is with lesser amounts—two to six drinks—that the risks remain imprecisely established at this time. Animal models of the FAS are being developed. They may assist in the determination of how much and when the drinking of alcoholic beverages is harmful to the fetus. Mice, rats, rabbits, and other species produce litters that show features of the FAS when on a diet that includes sufficient alcohol. Some of the embryos are so defective that resorption or spontaneous abortions occur.

ATYPICAL FAS VARIANTS

Milder variants of the FAS are probably common but are less often diagnosed. Children of heavily drinking parents may show borderline intelligence, behavioral problems, including minimal brain dysfunction (MBD), and poor learning ability. MBD is a significant clinical problem, and a certain number of these children could have derived their poor attention span and hyperkinetic behavior from a mother's alcoholism.

In a study at Washington University, 20 percent of the fathers and 5 percent of the mothers of MBD children were alcoholics. In the control group of nonhyperactive children only 10 percent of the fathers and none of the mothers were alcoholics. These findings have been confirmed in a subsequent UCLA study.

Another possible variant of the FAS is the child who is "slow in everything," "fails to thrive," or just looks "funny." Despite the dangers of overdiagnosing this condition, it is likely that the range of damage must extend from the fetus that is so disabled by alcohol that it is stillborn, through the readily diagnosed FAS infant, to the child with only minimal evidence of psychophysical impairment.

THE PROSPECTIVE STUDIES

Three major studies funded by the NIAAA are now exploring the relationship of alcohol to teratogenesis. In the Boston City Hospital survey, 74 percent of the infants born to women who imbibed more than 10 drinks a day demonstrated the FAS. In the Seattle (University of Washington) study, 12 percent of women who used two ounces of ethanol (about 4 to 5 drinks) a day delivered FAS children. Of 90 women who used less than two ounces of ethanol, two cases of FAS were found (2.2 percent).

From Loma Linda University and four cooperating Southern California hospitals, some preliminary results are available. Heavy alcohol users had more spontaneous abortions than moderate, low, or non-users. In fact, they had 10 times as many spontaneous abortions as non-users of alcohol. Other points emerging from this study are that heavy drinking is ordinarily associated with heavy smoking, greater coffee use, a tendency to use more drugs, and a tendency to eat junk foods.

In addition to these investigations, many other studies in animals and humans are underway. The newborn of a variety of animal species showed hyperactivity and poor learning ability when the mothers had received an adequate diet nutritionally plus alcohol that produced a blood level of 200-300 mg/dl.

PREVENTION

It seems clear that the FAS is a major cause of congenital mental and physical disorders. It is probably the most important preventable cause of birth defects. What is needed is an educational program aimed at the public, especially heavy-drinking women, and all physicians that will change our attitudes about drinking during pregnancy.

It was not uncommon in the past to recommend that expectant mothers take some wine or an alcohol-containing tonic before meals. Even this amount of ethanol may be undesirable, especially when combined with certain kinds of social drinking.

A bill has been introduced into the Congress that will require warning labels addressed to pregnant women on all alcoholic beverage containers (whiskey, wine, and beer) including alcohol-containing proprietary medicines.

Alcoholics should not conceive, and for those who do, termination of pregnancy should be available. If such women want to have a child, they should stop drinking before conception and throughout the pregnancy.

The developing information about the FAS combined with the increased prevalence of drinking by women, especially young women, requires that a special effect be made to make all of them aware of the potential for serious adverse effects upon the fetus.

SUMMARY

The FAS has an overall pattern of defects that are so similar from child to child that they are probably due to a single cause. The likelihood that the cause is alcohol's effect upon the maternal and fetal metabolism is great. The number of involved offspring increases as the amount of alcohol consumed by the mother increases; in other words, it is dose related. Alcohol crosses the placenta easily. In fact, it can be smelled at delivery in the amnionic fluid of women who have been drinking before or during labor. The developing tissues of the fetus are known to be more sensitive to the toxic effects of ethanol than are adult cellular structures.

This is a preventable condition with the responsibility placed on the woman who is or is about to become pregnant. In addition to the intense study of the role of the mother's alcohol use during pregnancy in inducing the FAS, it would be well to examine the role of the heavily drinking father prior to conception.

The reason why the medical profession has been lax in recommending abstinence from alcohol during pregnancy in the past is the residual notion that still pervades our thinking—that alcohol is not a drug.

CONCLUSION

If you drink, don't drive—or get pregnant.
If you get pregnant, drive—but don't drink.

REFERENCE

1. George, M.D. London life in the eighteenth century. New York, Capricorn, 1965 (Orig. 1925), p. 31.

BIBLIOGRAPHY

- Hanson, J.W., *et al*. Fetal alcohol syndrome: Experience with 41 patients. JAMA. 235:1458, 1976.
- Jones, K.L., *et al*. Pattern of malformation in offspring of chronic alcoholic mothers. Lancet. 1:1267, 1973.

- Jones, K.L., and Smith, D.W. Recognition of the fetal alcohol syndrome in early infancy. Lancet, 2:999, 1973.
- Jones, K.L., and Smith, D.W. The fetal alcohol syndrome. Teratology. 12:1, 1975.
- Ouellette, E.M., *et al.* Adverse effects on offspring of maternal alcohol abuse during pregnancy. New Engl. J. Med. 297:528, 1977.
- Shaywitz, B.A. Fetal alcohol syndrome: An ancient problem rediscovered. Drug Therapy (Hosp). 53–60 (Jan.) 1978.

5. Teenage Drinking: The Bottle Babies

Occasional drinking until drunk and restless behavior while intoxicated have been fairly conventional youthful activities associated with growing up in America.

Adolescents have imbibed both for the effects of the ethanol and for the symbolic meaning of the act of drinking. Partaking of our national intoxicant was often an effort at self-treatment for adolescent shyness and anxiety. Drinking has the double effect of producing and of justifying disinhibited acting-out behavior. The cultural symbolism of drinking by adolescents is that it simultaneously means "being one of the boys" (or girls) and "being a man," or "being grown up."

Youthful imbibing, then, directly derives from our cultural attitudes toward drinking. Although legally forbidden, drinking by those underage tends to be condoned or at least understood by most parents and authorities.

During the past few years the established mode has changed significantly. The following trends have been well documented:

1. Drinking during and out of school has extended down to grammar school students and is more frequently encountered than in the past.

2. Girls are increasingly involved in "ever having used" alcohol and in regularly drinking. By the time they graduate from high school as many girls as boys use alcoholic beverages, but not yet as often.

3. The combined use of alcohol and other drugs is often observed. Juvenile polydrug use with alcohol as the basic intoxicant is a growing problem.

4. Not only are more youngsters trying alcoholic beverages, but large

numbers are drinking heavily and consistently. Pubescent alcoholism has been diagnosed in a number of pediatric psychiatric clinics.

THE EXTENT

Most surveys agree that drinking starts earlier these days. The San Mateo school district survey, which has been taken yearly since 1968, indicates that any use of alcoholic beverages by 9-12th graders during the past year rose from 65 percent in 1968 to 86 percent in 1974. Male and female students using 10 or more times increased from 25 percent to 54 percent. For those using 50 or more times during the past year, the rate increased from 16 percent in 1970 to 29 percent in 1974. It should be pointed out that even the 1968–1970 rates were quite high when compared with student usage during the 1950s or earlier.

A national survey done in 1974 reported that 63 percent of boys and 54 percent of girls in the seventh grade have had a drink. By the time they reach the 12th grade this has increased to 93 percent of the boys and 87 percent of the girls. Drinking among school dropouts is greater than among those remaining in school. Therefore, teenage drinking is actually higher than reported from information collected from school populations. Six percent of high-school seniors drink daily.

Of course, the figures cited above do not necessarily represent excessive or problem drinking. Much of it was in a family setting taken with a meal or during special occasions. The only point that can be made from these data is that drinking has become more widespread during recent years. Abstinent young men and women are fewer in number even in sections of the country where they previously were numerous.

Because of our preoccupation with youthful drug abuse we have ignored the fact that in every survey, alcohol was the most frequently used and preferred drug. It is by far, the first mind-altering drug employed. Young people who do not use fermented beverages tend not to use other intoxicating drugs.

It is the practice of heavy binge drinking or of a consistent consumption of substantial amounts that is a matter for concern. Admittedly, patterns of drinking may be established during youth, and these can evolve into damaging drinking habits in later life. But problem adolescent drinking is a serious issue in its own right. When a young person has definite social, family, or health difficulties caused by his drinking, he can be considered a problem drinker.

The difficulty may occur in connection with an acute bout during which he becomes involved in a major auto accident. A series of drunk and disorderly arrests would indicate poor behavioral controls. Certainly, the chronic use of large amounts that leads to physical or psychological impairment, inability to attend to school work or a job, or impaired social relationships can be considered problem drinking. Many of the physical impairments of sustained, excessive alcohol intake are delayed (brain damage, liver failure, peripheral neuritis, etc.) so that only presumptive indications of future physical or neurological disability are possible.

THE ADOLESCENT ALCOHOLIC

Reports from the National Institute of Alcoholism and Alcohol Abuse confirm the rapid increase in heavy teenage drinking. Dr. M.E. Chafetz, ex-director of NIAAA, said that 5 percent of young Americans have a drinking problem. The estimated number of problem drinkers between the ages of 12 and 17 is 1.3 million, with 750,000 believed to be hard-core alcoholics. A Boston suburb study found that by age 18, 7 percent of the boys were problem drinkers. They had family, school, or police difficulties. If these estimates are correct, then the teenager is drinking just as unwisely as the adult, for 5 to 7 percent of adults are also in trouble with their alcohol usage.

"Drying out" centers report a staggering increase in teenage clients. One program in Houston has witnessed an increase in this age group from only 6 teenagers to 1,200 in three years. Eight- and nine-year-olds have been registered for alcohol detoxification in this and other clinics.

Alcoholics Anonymous (AA) has 27 groups for "teenagers and pre-teenagers" in Southern California alone. One report from New York City schools states that 10 percent of the junior and senior high school students are "already or potential alcoholics."

Many of the well-known signs of tissue damage by alcohol are not seen in pediatric alcoholics. These will come later. Gastritis and gastrointestinal hemorrhage, though, are present in the young and old alike. They are the result of stimulation of hydrochloric acid production and the retardation of acid absorption from the gastroduodenal tract. Inflammatory and ulcerative changes in the mucous membrane result. At Childrens Hospital in Los Angeles patients 12 to 20 years old with alcohol-related ailments like gastritis and internal bleeding are not uncommon.

Among military personnel at the San Diego Naval Hospital, alcoholics had a death rate of 15 per 1,000 patients a year. This compares with a rate of two per 1,000 for naval and 10 per 1,000 for marine personnel. The major causes of death among the alcoholics were suicide, accidents, cirrhosis of the liver, pancreatitis, and peptic ulcer. When it is recalled that diseases like pancreatitis and cirrhosis do not become manifest until after many years of steady drinking, death in the 30s means a very early onset of excessive use.

It is behavioral toxicity that dominates the picture of problem drinking by teenagers. Recurrent truancy, family disruptions, and illegal activities are the presenting signs. The stealing of beer, wine, and saleable items is well known. The suburban form of this activity is called "garaging." Rowdy group drinking parties, some of which culminate in the use of dangerous weapons, are regularly reported in the press. Intoxicated youngsters are apt to become involved in malicious mischief in schools, parks, and unoccupied dwellings. The arrest rate for intoxication in those under 18 has tripled during the past decade. Accidental death, a leading cause of lethality in this age group, is particularly frequent among adolescent imbibers. A third to a half of all accidents is associated with drinking.

ALCOHOL AND DRIVING

A considerable controversy centers on the effects of lowering the legal drinking age in some states and the incidence of car accidents. In Michigan during the first year that 18-year-olds could legally buy alcoholic beverages, the auto accident rate for those 18 to 20 years old increased by 119 percent. Arrests in New Jersey rose 60 percent.

On one side of the argument are those who say that these statistics merely reflect normal yearly increases and the differential treatment accorded young drivers by the police. Others view these figures more seriously and believe that young people will die or be injured on the highways at a rate far exceeding the worst years of the Viet Nam conflict.

Sixty percent of those killed in drunk driving accidents are in their teens. Even in a single year the jump in alcohol-related accidents is impressive. The California Highway Patrol reported that deaths in the 12 to 20 age group rose from 268 in 1973 to 375 in 1974. Traffic injuries rose from 4,499 in 1973 to 6,252 in 1974.

FACTORS CONTRIBUTING TO PROBLEM DRINKING

Earlier studies emphasized the family unit as the place where lifelong drinking practices are formed. This was probably true when families exerted a considerable influence on adolescent development. It may be somewhat less valid at present. The parent's drinking behavior remains an important predictor of the teenager's drinking habits. Drinking parents ordinarily will have drinking children with the degree of usage reflecting parental patterns. Abstinent parents are more likely to have abstinent children. Of course many exceptions exist. Some children will be so upset by a drunken parent that they will react by abstaining. Overly strict, teetotalling parents may alienate a child, causing a complete rejection of the parental prohibitions. These children seem prone to use liquor intemperately.

In recent years more emphasis is being placed on the influence of peers. Heavy drinking often starts on playgrounds, street corners, and similar youth gathering areas. Drinking at school special events and athletic contests has occasionally terminated in riots and forced a cancellation of the event.

Whether a child will drink, and how he will behave if drunk, is strongly determined by the culture. It is the culture or subculture that provides cues through family, friends, or mass media and informs the youth as to what is permitted. In certain subcultures aggressiveness while drunk is considered normal behavior.

The individual's personality is also a determinant in the development of destructive drinking practices. At times it is difficult to determine whether certain personality features cause or are the result of drinking excessively. Diminished personal controls, impulsivity, and antisocial trends are supposed to be predisposing personality factors. It may be so, but it should be remembered that alcohol intoxication also releases such behavior.

Young people with personality deficits in the area of mood and ego controls do tend to seek out alcohol in order to deal with their noxious feelings and instability. If drinking dissolves their problems, then they are later inclined to use it often and in large amounts. Not all youthful problem drinkers have a major personality defect. They may be relatively intact psychologically, but might have become overinvolved because the practice happened to be a cultural or family norm.

BEVERAGE CHOICE

Beer is popular among young drinkers. Although it is a dilute alcohol solution, beer is capable of causing all the problems of stronger drink. The new sweet ''pop'' wines are a growing favorite. Beer cans and wine bottles have become a litter problem in some schoolyards, parking lots, and beaches frequented by youths. Another contender for favor is the vodka mixes like Orange Fling and Strawberry Fling sold in bottles that resemble soda pop bottles. When liquor is used, it is often in the form of vodka because it is cheap, blends with the mix, and is less detectable on the breath.

ALCOHOL AND OTHER DRUGS

The earlier prediction that the juvenile use of cannabis would lead to a reduction in alcohol consumption has not been realized. On the contrary, marihuana users drink more alcohol than nonmarihuana users. They are used separately and together. In the latter instance it is believed that marihuana has synergistic sedative effects with alcohol. When a inquiry is made into which mind altering drug was used first, the answer is generally the legal ones: alcohol and tobacco. Later, marihuana and other drugs are added.

It is understandable that alcoholic drinks would be the preferred intoxicants.

They are less expensive, more readily available, and less illegal than others. They cover up the fact that illicit drugs were also used. Parents are, somehow, relieved to find their children have been "stoned" on alcohol rather than a nonalcoholic substance.

Ethanol is here to stay. A recent survey of 200 drug abuse agencies reported that the teenage use of alcohol and marihuana was increasing, while other abused agents were decreasing slightly or were unchanged. The combined ingestion of alcohol along with other central nervous system depressants will reinforce the depressant effect. This would be true for sedatives, hypnotics, narcotics, anesthetics, and tranquilizers. When consumed with stimulants or hallucinogens, the result will be a reduction in the stimulant effect or an aberrant, unpredictable reaction.

PREVENTION

To prevent the overindulgence of a culturally entrenched, ubiquitous substance like alcohol hardly seems possible. It is especially difficult because our pattern of usage does not condemn, and sometimes applauds, excessive drinking. This is the message our children perceive, over and over, verbally and nonverbally.

What can be done? First of all, the adolescent abstainer should be reinforced and made to feel that his decision is sensible, and even courageous because it goes counter to the popular mode. But in a society pervaded by alcohol, in which it is a symbol for hospitality, fun, sexuality, and maturity, most young people are unable to swim against the alcoholic flood.

Exhorting them to renounce drink will rarely work. Instead of proscribing alcohol intake, its use should be wisely prescribed. Children should learn responsible drinking, moderation should be stressed, and drunkenness condemned from the parents in words and deeds. An episode of drunkenness that results in the destruction of property, injury, or in passing out should be met with firm disapproval. Unfortunately, such behavior is often overtly or covertly reinforced.

TREATMENT

The management of teenage alcohol abuse is by no means easy or invariably successful. It is difficult for the youngster to identify that he is doing something harmful or that he is sick. Many of those around him, young and old, seem to be drinking as he is. Even if he admits he has a problem, his motivation to correct it is often less than adequate. He may sample an AA meeting without committing himself. If pushed to go to a psychiatrist or other mental health worker, he tends to drop out of treatment rather quickly.

Groups of teenagers with similar problems led by an understanding therapist can be helpful for some. Teenage AA assists those who are willing to accept the program. Religious appeals will attract certain youths. Some exploratory methods show promise, including one which trains appropriate teenage counselors who, with back-up assistance, may be more acceptable to the alcoholic adolescent. At times, medical counseling and psychiatric referral is mandatory, particularly in emotionally disturbed youngsters. Behavior modification has not been tried often enough in this group to comment on it. Antabuse therapy is not indicated in young people except, perhaps, in a special military situation.

Family therapy is sometimes the treatment of choice, for example, when family pressures are laid on the young person whose drinking is in response to a pathological family situation. A foster family may be needed when one or both parents are alcoholics. It is clear that the young person cannot return to his group of heavily drinking friends should he succeed in moderating or halting his use of alcohol.

6. Lowering the Drinking Age: Effects on Auto Accidents

A move to amend the law to permit 18-year-olds to vote and enter into legal contracts started 15 years ago. It then seemed anomalous to treat 18 and 20-year-olds as adults and not permit them to drink alcoholic beverages legally.

Therefore, between 1970 and 1973 about half of the United States and all 10 of the Canadian provinces and two territories lowered the legal drinking age. Some jurisdictions lowered the age to 18, others to 19. It should be noted that the legal drinking age has been 18 in New York since 1934 and 18 in Louisiana since 1948.

The legislation was viewed as enlightened and forward-looking. It was believed that if consuming alcohol would lose the symbolic significance of being grown-up, young people might learn to drink moderately and more wisely than their elders. Furthermore, most teenagers had been drinking anyway, despite their inability to purchase alcoholic beverages.

Because of restrictions on purchase and possession the patterns of their usage may have encouraged them to drink rapidly and excessively. The hope existed that the accident rate for the under-21-year-olds might even decrease since the 18-year-old in Connecticut, for example, would not have to drive to New York to purchase and consume alcohol before driving back home.

Drivers under 21 tended to have high rates of automobile collisions even before the legal drinking age was lowered. Their driving records have been poorer than older drivers, and auto insurance rates reflect this data. Even when unimpaired by the effects of alcohol, they do not drive as safely as older drivers. Sixteen and 17-year-olds perform worse than 18 and 19-year-olds insofar as accident rates are concerned. Why this should be is not precisely known. It is suggested that less caution and prudence in driving are characteristic of some young drivers. In addition, it may take years before the reflexes for successful and safe driving are fully developed.

In attempting to explain why only young drivers as a group have a high accident involvement, Carlson points out that they are faced with two learning situations: how to drive, and how to drive after drinking.(9) These two simultaneous learning situations result in a higher crash involvement than could be explained by the amount of time they spend on the road.

The disproportionately high crash statistics correlate with night driving, which he regards as the most important variable second only to the blood alcohol concentration. The overrepresentation of youth in the group of fatally injured drivers, both with or without alcohol, is partly attributable to their life-style, which includes night driving for recreational purposes.

DRINKING AND DRIVING

The effects of lowering the drinking age on various types of car accidents have been examined in numerous studies. They were intensively studied in Michigan, where police statistics were analyzed shortly after the law changed. An increase of 119 percent in alcohol-related collisions among 18 to 20-year-olds was found when prelaw and postlaw periods were compared.(1) By comparison, older drivers showed a 14 percent increase in the same time period.

In another study, the rate of alcohol-related fatal accidents was compared for those over 21 and for persons 18 to 20 years of age.(2) Those older than 21 showed a 9 percent increase for the first six months and an 8 percent increase for the second six months after the law change. The 18 to 20-year-olds showed an 88 percent increase during the first six months and a 13 percent increase during the second six months. This study provided some hope that the problem was self-limiting and merely reflected an initial reckless attitude about drinking and driving.

In fact, Zylman attributed the changes to the normal cyclic fluctuations of such data and to the pressure on the police to report alcohol involvement in younger drivers who were in collisions.(3) This does not seem to be the case, as further studies have been reported.

Reports from other states support the hypothesis that significant increases in driving accidents occur among 18 to 20-year-olds in states where the drinking age was lowered in comparison to the same age group in states that did not change their legislation. (4,5) This is especially true for single vehicle accidents involving males between the hours of 9 p.m. and 3 a.m., a pattern that is known to be associated with drinking drivers in a majority of instances. The number of alcohol-related vehicle crashes involving young women is only about 10 percent of those involving young men. Their accident rate has not risen as steeply.

In Canada the experience has been approximately the same. An Ontario study showed that drivers 16 to 19 years of age were the only group who showed a significant increase in all types of collisions during the six months after the law change compared to the half year before.(6)

Whitehead investigated police records in London, Ontario for three years before and two years after the driving law change.(7) He gathered data on drivers involved in collisions who were from 16 to 20 and those 24 years of age. From these age groups he had a nonlegal drinking group (16 to 17), the newly legal drinking group (18 to 20), and a legal drinking young adult comparison (24) group that had not been affected by the new law.

The results showed increases in alcohol-associated accidents during the postlaw period. Increases of more than 300 percent were found for the 18 and 19-year-olds and more than 150 percent for the 20-year-olds. The 24-year-olds had an increase of only 20 percent during the same period. Whitehead considered the possibility that the police were especially diligent in reporting alcohol-related accidents among young drivers, but he rejected the assumption on the basis of multiple lines of evidence. The fact that the second year record was no better than the first postlaw year indicates that the problem is not simply a transient "release from restraint" effect that subsides in time.

In an extension of the study during an additional two years, Whitehead provided longer-term information.(8) He detected a "spillover effect" of the law on 16 and 17-year-olds . Whereas the incidence of alcohol-associated accidents rose immediately after the law went into effect in the 18 to 20-year-old group, the increase was delayed until the second year in the 16 to 17-year-old group. This might be explained by the extra time needed for the diffusion of the awareness of the easier access to alcoholic beverages to the younger age group. Many high school seniors are 18 years old and they are a readily available source of beverages for their younger friends.

It might be argued that an upsurge in alcohol use is occurring among youth and that regardless of lowering the legal purchase age, the increase in car accidents would have occurred anyway. This factor may account for some of the increase. The abruptness of the change, however, after passage of the alcohol-purchasing age law for the 18 to 20-year-olds is persuasive that the law was an important causal factor.

DISCUSSION

It is not easy to eradicate a behavior in an individual or in a society once it has been established. The disappointing increase in car accidents among drivers under 21 after passage of legislation reducing the drinking age indicates that 20 or 21 may be a more satisfactory age than 18 or 19 for permitting purchase of alcohol-containing beverages.

Some governments recently have begun to raise their minimum age for drinking and others are considering such a course. Maine has reversed its laws and changed the drinking age from 18 to 20. Saskatchewan has raised it from 18 to 19. It is difficult to say whether the upward revision of the minimum age will reverse the accident rate. Meanwhile, other jurisdictions, including California, are going ahead with proposals to lower the age from 21 for the legal purchase of alcoholic beverages.

Other proposals to deter excessive drinking include: (1) issuance of provisional driver's licenses to the 18 to 20 age group to be withdrawn for any moving violation, (2) raising the tax on beverages to increase their cost, and (3) augmenting the spot testing of the driver's breath for alcohol quantity at the roadside to deter drinking before or during the operation of a vehicle.

It is not easy to be optimistic about reversing the current high level of automobile accidents in younger men. Secondary prevention through identification of those at high risk of dysfunctional drinking-driving and their education in the hope that they will improve their drinking or their driving has not yet been proven to be effective in the age group under consideration. Efforts such as driving under the influence (DUI) programs directed at teenage violators have not reported their followup statistics.

It is in primary prevention—education and learning by example of young children to drink moderately or not at all—that the best hopes lie. This approach is a long-term effect and cannot be expected to produce any impact until a generation or two has elapsed. It also means that adult drinking patterns will have to moderate and that will be a formidable task.

Furthermore, it means that driving motor vehicles will have to be considered a complex operation needing the highest level of sober skill to operate safely. Such cultural value shifts are required before any fundamental changes can take place in our highway behavior.

Can such value shifts occur? They are possible, but the answer is in doubt.

REFERENCES

1. Hammond, R.L. Legal drinking age at 18 or 21: Does it make a difference? *J. Alcohol Drug Education.* 18:9–13, 1973.
2. MICAP RECAP. Report No. 35 Michigan Council on Alcohol Problems, Lansing, Mi. 1973.
3. Zylman, R. Fatal crashes among Michigan youth following reduction of legal drinking age. *Quart. J. Stud. Alcohol.* 35:283–286, 1974.
4. Williams, P.H., *et al.* The legal minimum drinking age and fatal motor vehicle crashes. *J. Legal Studies.* 4:219–239, 1975.
5. Cucchiario, S. *et al.* The effect of the 18 year old drinking age on auto accidents. Massachusetts Institute of Technology Operations Research Center, Cambridge, Ma. 1974.

6. Schmidt, W. and Kornaczewski, A. L'abaissement de l'age auquel-la loide l' Ontario permit d'absorber de l'alcool et ses effets sur les accidents de'automobile attribuales a l'alcool. *Toxicomanies.* 8:105–116, 1975.
7. Whitehead, P.C. *et al.* Change in the drinking age: Impact on young drivers. *J. Stud. Alcohol.* 36:1209–1223, 1975.
8. Whitehead, P.C. Alcohol and young drivers. Impact and implications of lowering the drinking age. Non-Medical Use of Drugs Directorate, Department of National Health and Welfare, Monograph Series No. 1.,1977.
9. Carlson, W.L. Age exposure and alcohol involvement in night crashes. *J. Safety Research.* 5:247, 1973.

7. The Oriental Syndrome

A large number of Orientals have a sensitivity to alcoholic beverages that is manifested by a marked facial flush shortly after consuming even small amounts. Some American Indians, East Europeans, and members of other cultures may show a similar hypersensitivity to ethanol. As little as one drink might bring on the temporary reddening of the face, neck, and, sometimes, the upper chest.

Along with the dilation of the skin capillaries, some highly sensitive individuals, or those who imbibe large amounts of alcohol, manifest additional autonomic symptoms. Hypotension, tachycardia, and bronchoconstriction can occur, and the person may feel exceedingly uncomfortable.

The flush may vary from a mild reddening of the skin around the mouth to severe flushing over the upper third of the body. Symptoms like dizziness, sleepiness, pounding in the head, and nausea are apt to accompany the cutaneous manifestations. Orientals who do not flush may experience certain of these generalized symptoms more often than non-Orientals after equivalent amounts of alcohol.

The flush syndrome has been cited as an important reason why the incidence of alcoholism in Orientals may be lower than that of other races. Of course, other factors must play important roles, but the inability to drink large amounts comfortably may reinforce sociocultural influences.

Those who exhibit the flush syndrome tend to be either abstainers or modest drinkers due to their physiologic intolerance. Large quantities, however, are taken by some sensitive individuals who run the risk of asthmatic attacks or cardiovascular collapse. The problems that a number of American Indians have with excessive drinking points out that physiologic discomfort is not necessarily a bar to heavy alcohol consumption. Actually, no investigation has been done to determine whether Indian flushers are less likely to consume large amounts of alcoholic beverages than non-flushing Indians.

ETIOLOGY

The precise cause of this aberration of alcohol metabolism is unknown but a genetic component is undoubtedly involved. It has been assumed that a reduction or an absence of the enzyme aldehyde dehydrogenase produces a retention of acetaldehyde. Acetaldehyde is the first metabolic product of alcohol and is much more toxic than ethanol itself. The accumulation of acetaldehyde in the body could account for the unpleasant symptoms of the Oriental flush syndrome. Although flushers have higher blood acetaldehyde levels than non-flushers, the elevation is not marked, and acetaldehyde may not be a complete explanation of the phenomenon. The release of biogenic amines like norepinephrine, histamine, and serotonin also occurs, but these might be the result of the stressful flush reaction rather than a cause of it.

ANTABUSE AND RELATED DRUGS

It is well established that disulfiram (Antabuse) and other alcohol-sensitizing drugs increase blood acetaldehyde levels due to an inhibition of aldehyde dehydrogenase. Other compounds that act in a like manner, although not as efficiently, are citrated calcium carbamide (Temposil) and sulfonylurea compounds like Orinase.

The symptoms of the alcohol-Antabuse reaction are rather similar to the flush syndrome, but may be more intense depending on the alcohol and the Antabuse dosages. The *Physicians Desk Reference*(1) describes the reaction as follows: "flushing, throbbing in head and neck, throbbing headache, respiratory difficulty, nausea, copious vomiting, sweating, thirst, chest pain, palpitation, dyspnea, hyperventilation, tachycardia, hypotension, marked uneasiness, weakness, vertigo, blurred vision and confusion. In severe reactions there may be respiratory depression, cardiovascular collapse, myocardial infarction, acute congestive heart failure, unconsciousness, convulsions and death."

It has been speculated that alcohol-sensitive persons have a built-in alcohol-Antabuse situation that should protect them from overdrinking, but it does not always do so. Patients on Antabuse have deliberately challenged its deterrent effect on occasion by drinking alcohol. Some people will drink wood alcohol, rubbing alcohol, fusel oil, and other toxic concoctions indicating that pleasurable effects are not a requirement for drinking intoxicants, nor are noxious effects a bar. Apparently the rewards of intoxication outweigh the aversive effects for these people.

ACETALDEHYDE

Acetaldehyde has been accused of much of the toxic impact of heavy alcohol consumption. For example, the hangovers, alcoholic cardiomyopathy, alcoholic liver injury, and impaired protein synthesis in alcoholics have been related to acetaldehyde. These assumptions are based upon the fact that acetaldehyde is 10 to 20 times more toxic than ethyl alcohol. No evidence for a fetal acetaldehyde syndrome has been claimed, perhaps because the placenta is very efficient in oxidizing acetaldehyde to acetate.

The problem is that although acetaldehyde can induce most of the symptoms of the flush syndrome, it does so at blood levels higher than those found in people who are flushing. The suggestion has been made that flushing might be produced by the high initial spike of acetaldehyde production a few minutes after alcohol intake. This may take place due to a surge of ethanol transformation to acetaldehyde because of a highly active alcohol dehydrogenase—as has been commonly found in the Japanese population.(2)

Thus the flush response could be caused by a relative decrease in the activity of acetaldehye dehydrogenase or a relative increase in the activity of alcohol dehydrogenase. A third possibility is that the end organs (the skin capillaries over the blush area) are highly sensitive to ordinary amounts of acetaldehyde.

Animal studies have shown that compounds that produce an accumulation of acetaldehyde in the organism will cause the animals to restrict their drinking in a free-choice situation. Furthermore, the differences in alcohol consumption between genetically different strains of mice are directly related to differences in the way that they metabolize alcohol and acetaldehyde.

HISTAMINE

Another chemical candidate for the genesis of the flush response is histamine. As will be indicated, alcohol-sensitive people can develop hives over the blush area. This may be modulated by a release of histamine that dilates the skin capillaries and increases their permeability. Histamine is known to produce headache (histamine headache), a pulsating fullness in the head, bronchoconstriction, tachycardia, and hypotension (anaphylactic shock). Despite the overlap of symptoms, there is a little proof that histamine release is the primary cause of the flush syndrome.

RESEARCH STUDIES

In one study(3), 55 Chinese and Japanese men swallowed about one ounce of ethanol (0.4 ml/kg) in a 19 percent solution. Thirty-three (60 percent) developed a cutaneous flush, some of them had hives. Of 11 Caucasians, only one (9 percent) flushed; and the flush was noted to be mild. The only highly significant biochemical difference between flushers and non-flushers was a lower serum hydrocortisone level in the former group.

The decreased hydrocortisone response among Orientals as compared to Occidentals was also significant, but this was seen as a secondary effect of the exposure to the flush provocation test. In this study, the mean acetaldehyde blood level of all Orientals was higher than among the Occidentals (p < .05) 30 minutes after drinking alcohol. Plasma histamine levels were not detectable in either group, nor were skin tests for alcohol positive.

Ewing and his colleagues(4) reported that in 24 persons of Oriental parentage, 17 (70 percent) showed a facial flush following alcohol intake. In 24 Caucasian men and women, three (12.5 percent) demonstrated a flush. Capillary blood flow to the skin increased in the flushers; some had drops in systolic blood pressure in excess of 10 mm Hg. A mild tachycardia was recorded. Symptoms such as pounding in the head, muscle weakness, and dizziness were mentioned. Many more Orientals reported family members who flushed than did Occidental subjects.

A study(5) that compared 656 Chinese, 654 Japanese, 444 Hapa Haoles (one Oriental and one Caucasian parent), and 674 Caucasians, all living in Hawaii, revealed a much larger proportion of Orientals who flushed after drinking. Hapa Haoles had approximately the same percentage of flushers as the Oriental group. A greater percentage of Orientals reported no use of alcohol, possibly because of the unpleasant reaction. Caucasians drank much more, and Hapa Haoles were intermediate in their alcohol consumption.

American Indians also have a higher rate of flushing than do people of European extraction, according to Wolff.(6) This is quite reasonable in view of the Mongoloid derivation of the Amerindians and their prehistoric migration across the Bering Strait. Fifty Caucasoids, 30 Cree Indians, 20 half-Mongoloid/half-Caucasoids, 15 Americans of Chinese or Japanese origin, and a small number of one-quarter-Mongoloid/three-quarters-Caucasoids were tested with an alcohol challenge. Visible flushing appeared in 4 percent of the Caucasoids, 50 percent of the Indians, 80 percent of the pure Orientals, 90 percent of those with half-Mongoloid ancestry, and 75 percent of those of one-quarter-Mongoloid extraction. The flush appeared within a few minutes. No male-female differences were noted. It would seem that the genotype for flushing is a dominant, since quarter- and half-Mongoloids inherit the trait in a high proportion of instances. In order to eliminate a placebo response, some of those who flushed after oral alcoholic beverages were administered either an alcohol solution or saline intravenously. Flushing occured only when the alcohol was injected.

Wolff also reported that when tiny amounts of port wine in a glucose solution were given to Oriental infants, 74 percent flushed. The same preparation caused flushing in only five percent of Occidental infants. He concluded that dietary or cultural factors did not account for the differences between Orientals and Occidentals.

Twenty-six Japanese were given 200 ml of sake (a wine made of fermented rice) during a 10-minute period. Of these, 11 flushed, and 15 did not. Those who flushed had a significantly higher acetaldehyde blood level than those who did not. This is contrary to a number of studies that reported no relationship between acetaldehyde level and flushing.

SUMMARY

Many people of Mongolian ancestry metabolize alcohol in a manner that produces flushing and sometimes physiologic symptoms. This does not seem to protect many of them from excessive drinking since the rates of alcoholism have increased, particularly in Japan.(7) Furthermore, the American Indians who share the flush response because of their Mongolian lineage also have substantial problems with alcohol consumption.

REFERENCES

1. *Physicians Desk Reference*, 33rd Edition, Medical Economics Co., Oradell, NJ, 1979, p. 594.
2. Lundros, K.O. Acetaldehyde—Its metabolism and role in the actions of alcohol. In: *Research Advances in Alcohol and Drug Problems*, Vol. II. Ed.: Israel, Y., *et al.*, Plenum, New York, 1978, pp. 111–176.
3. Seto, H., *et al.* Biochemical correlates of ethanol-induced flushing in Orientals. *J. Stud. Alcohol.* 39:1–11, 1978.
4. Ewing, J.A., *et al.* Alcohol sensitivity and ethnic background. *Am. J. Psychiatry.* 131:206–210, 1974.
5. Wilson, J.R., *et al.* Ethnic variation in use and effects of alcohol. *Drug & Alcohol Dependence.* 3:147–151, 1978.
6. *Wolff, P.H.* Vasomotor sensitivity to alcohol in diverse mongoloid populations. *Am. J. Human Genetics.* 25:193–199, 1973.
7. Mendelson, J.G. and Mello, N.K. Biologic Concomitants of Alcoholism. *New England Journal of Medicine.* 301:912, 1979.

8. Alcoholic Hypoglycemia

Hypoglycemia is both an overdiagnosed and underdiagnosed condition. Since many of the symptoms resemble an anxiety attack or other sort of "nervous" reaction, the two conditions may be misidentified with each other.

It is not surprising that hypoglycemia presents with symptoms of anxiety. As blood sugar levels drop, adrenalin secretion is stimulated, producing a mobilization of glycogen stores with an increased availability of glucose. Adrenalin also causes tenseness, sweating, faintness, hunger, tachycardia, and tremulousness.

Other evidences of hypoglycemia are due to the cortical depression from a very low blood sugar, and they include confusion, visual disturbances, ataxia, headache, muscle weakness, convulsions, and coma. A fasting blood sugar level of 40 mg percent or under and a rapid response to intravenous or oral sugar are confirmatory diagnostic evidence. Sometimes a 3- or 5-hour glucose tolerance test is needed to provoke low blood sugar levels when the patient is seen between attacks. In severe cases the blood sugar level has dropped to as low as 5 mg percent.

ALCOHOL AND HYPOGLYCEMIA

The causes of hypoglycemia are many (see Table 8-1), but the focus here is on the relationships between alcohol consumption and hypoglycemic episodes. One report estimates that 70 percent of all reactive hypoglycemias are induced by alcohol. Some of the symptoms mentioned are reminiscent of certain alcoholic states. For example, the acute intoxicated condition, the delirium tremens, and chronic inebriation all may resemble some of the manifestations of hypoglycemia. Stupor and coma in a person who has been drinking must be quickly differentiated because, untreated, extremely low blood sugar levels are incompatible with survival. People whose autonomic or neurologic symptoms and signs exceed the amount of ethyl alcohol consumed should be suspected of having hypoglycemia.

Even the sober, convalescent alcoholic may have a low blood sugar level. During sobriety he may still have an unstable glucose-regulating mechanism that produces weakness, headache, a rapid pulse, sweating, hunger feelings, and anxiety. This usually occurs many hours after a carbohydrate-rich meal, and is associated with a craving for coffee, sweets, and soft drinks. Unless the distressing symptoms are brought under control, they may provoke a relapse.

ALCOHOLIC HYPOGLYCEMIA: MECHANISMS

Alcohol ingestion does many things to carbohydrate metabolism, some of which culminate in reduced levels of circulating glucose. In healthy drinkers small amounts of alcohol produce a mild initial hyperglycemia—possibly because of the carbohydrate-sparing effect of the drug or because of alcohol's release of catecholamines that provoke glycogenolysis (liver glycogen breakdown to glucose). The elevated circulating glucose stimulates the beta cells of the pancreas to secrete insulin. If the person is sensitive to the glucose-lowering effects of insulin, mild hypoglycemia could result.

What is more common is that malnourished or fasting drinkers whose glycogen stores are greatly depleted will experience hypoglycemia even in the absence of liver disease. The hypoglycemic episode typically occurs after 4 or more hours of drinking. Since glucose and glycogen are readily manufactured from proteins and fats, it is apparent that gluconeogenesis (the synthesis of glucose from amino acids in protein and glycerol in fat) is also adversely affected by alcohol. This occurs because in the metabolism of alcohol, acetaldehyde and hydrogen ions are produced. The latter are immediately bound to NAD (nicotinamide adenine dinucleotide) to form $NADH_2$. The $NADH_2$ drives the chemical reactions toward lactate and away from the precursors of carbohydrate, like pyruvate.

Severe alcoholic liver damage can compound the distortions of carbohydrate metabolism. Glycogen is poorly stored in necrotic hepatocytes. But hypoglycemia occurs only in end stage cirrhosis. More commonly, hyperglycemia and frank diabetes develops as a result of alcoholic hepatitis and cirrhosis. This is attributed to a resistance to circulating insulin and is detectable in glucose and insulin tolerance tests. Insulin resistance may be secondary to increased amounts of circulating growth hormone, an insulin antagonist known to be elevated in cirrhotics. Chronic alcoholic pancreatitis also will cause diabetes, and this complication is evidently induced by diminished insulin production by the beta cells.

Table 8-1

The Differential Diagnosis of Hypoglycemia

I. Exogenous (Reactive) Causes

A. High intake or rapid absorption of carbohydrate
1. Insulin overshoot hypoglycemia
2. Postgastrectomy syndrome (dumping syndrome)

B. Inhibition of glycogenolysis by specific nutrients
1. Fructose intolerance
2. Galactosemia
3. Leucine sensitivity (maple syrup urine disease)

C. Drugs
1. Excess glucose utilization
   a. Excessive insulin administration
   b. Insulin effect intensified by propanolol, oxytetracyline, EDTA, manganese, etc.
   c. Excessive sulfonurea administration
   d. Sulfonurea effect intensified by sulfa drugs dicumarol, phenylbutazone, and alcohol
   e. Excess phenformin administration
2. Deficient glucose production
   a. Alcohol
   b. Salicylates
   c. Aminobenzoic acid
   d. Chlorpromazine
   e. Haloperidol
   f. Propoxyphene

II. Endogenous (Spontaneous) Causes

A. Excess glucose utilization
1. Insulinoma (tumor of pancreatic beta cells)
2. Deficiency of anti-insulin hormones: glucagon, cortisol, epinephrine, growth and thyroid hormones
3. Neonatal hypoglycemia of infants born of diabetic mothers

B. Excessive glucose utilization or excretion
1. Exercise
2. Fever
3. Pregnancy
4. Renal glycosuria
5. Certain tumors may utilize large amounts of glucose

C. Deficient glucose production
1. Liver disease
2. Glycogen mobilization disorder (glycogen storage diseases)
3. Glucose-6-phosphate deficiency (poor glucose release)
4. Fructose-1-6-diphosphotase deficiency

45

Pathologic drinking practices eventually will affect the intestine's ability to absorb carbohydrates and other nutrients by damage to the mucosa and deficiencies of the digestive enzymes of the pancreas. This end effect is similar to starvation or malnutrition, a contributory factor to hypoglycemia. Gastritis, associated with anorexia and vomiting, and the steatorrhea of the malabsorption syndrome also reduce carbohydrate absorption.

PREVENTION AND TREATMENT

Not only can severe hypoglycemia end fatally, but recurrent attacks can result in brain injury since glucose is the nerve cell's only nutritional substrate. Therefore, the termination and correction of such attacks are important. For those who sustain hypoglycemic episodes in connection with their alcohol use, abstention or a marked reduction in the amount consumed is strongly recommended. This step alone may eliminate the problem. If it does not, 4 to 6 small meals daily should be eaten. They should be low in carbohydrates and high in fat and protein in order not to stimulate insulin release. Caffeine is interdicted by some physicians for the same reason. For the acute attack, intravenous glucose is necessary if the patient cannot swallow. Fruit juices with added sugar are generally given by mouth to those whose symptoms are not severe.

Hypoglycemia is another reason why drinkers should not drive. The confusion, faintness, dizziness, and impaired psychomotor skills can lead to driving mishaps. If an incident that can be identified as hypoglycemia occurs while driving, the individual should pull over and stop as soon as it is safely possible. He should obtain some sugar-containing food and consume it. Relief ought to be noticeable within 10 minutes. People who have experienced a number of attacks usually keep a few chocolate bars in the glove compartment.

SUMMARY

When the symptoms of people who have been drinking exceed what would be expected from their blood alcohol concentration, hypoglycemia is one of the possibilities that should be considered. This is especially true in instances of coma associated with the consumption of alcoholic beverages. Those who have experienced hypoglycemic attacks while sober are well advised to avoid over-indulgence in ethanol. Drinkers who sustain such episodes ought to be cautioned to abstain or reduce their intake markedly.

Physicians must always consider the possibility of hypoglycemic stupor or coma in an unconscious person smelling of alcohol. A trial injection of glucose might be indicated as a diagnostic aid. People with insulin-producing tumors and with alcohol on their breath have been labelled drunks because of the bizarre behavior evoked by their very low blood sugar.

High alcohol intake can produce the following carbohydrate shifts and cause hypoglycemia:

1. decreased intake or loss of nutrients,

2. impaired absorption of carbohydrates and vitamins needed for carbohydrate metabolism,

3. diversion of pyruvate to lactate, preventing gluconeogenesis,

4. reduction of liver glycogen stores,

5. indirect stimulation of insulin secretion.

BIBLIOGRAPHY

- Baruh, S., *et al.* Fasting hypoglycemia. Med. Clin. N. Amer. 57:1441–1462, 1973.
- Cohen, S., A review of hypoglycemia and alcoholism with or without liver disease. Ann. N.Y. Acad. Sci. 273:338–342, 1976.
- Jaffe, B., *et al.* Hormonal response in ethanol-induced hypoglycemia. J. Studies Alcohol. 36:550–554, 1975.
- Kissin, B. & Begleiter, H. *The Biology of Alcoholism*, Vol. 1:Biochemistry. Plenum. N.Y., 1971.
- Leggett, J. & Favazza, A.R. Hypoglycemia: An overview. J. Clin. Psychiat. 39:51–57, 1978.
- Nikkola, E.A. & Taskinen, M.R. Ethanol-induced alterations of glucose tolerance, postglucose hypoglycemia and insulin secretion. Diabetes. 24:933–943, 1975.
- Ragnar, H., *et al.* Does a disturbed insulin release promote hypoglycemia in alcoholics? Acta. Med. Scand. 204:57–60, 1978.
- Searle, G., *et al.* Evaluation of ethanol hypoglycemia in man. Metabolism. 23:1023–1025, 1974.

9. Pathological Intoxication

Pathological intoxication—or alcohol idosyncratic intoxication, as it is called in DSM III—is a rather infrequent condition. But when a case is seen, it remains in the memory of those nearby because of the impressive panic or rage reactions. An older name for the disorder is *mania ā potu*. This term should be discarded because it has also been used in connection with the delirium tremens.

CLINICAL FEATURES

The essential characteristic is a marked behavioral change, usually in the direction of inappropriate belligerence and assaultiveness following the ingestion of a small quantity of alcoholic beverages. The amount consumed may be as little as one drink, but sometimes larger amounts are required to evoke the condition. However, it is not a quantity sufficient to produce intoxication. The behavior represents a marked change from the person's usual comportment.

The mental state reflects the unpredictable and destructive behavioral pattern. Confusion and disorganization of thought processes are evident. Speech is either incoherent or based on delusional thinking. It is the explosive fury in connection with the consumption of less than intoxicating amounts of alcohol that is most impressive. The rage reaction can result in serious injury to relatives, friends, or strangers. Homicides are a possibility, and a few serious suicide attempts have been reported. The condition terminates in a deep sleep. Upon awakening the person experiences a total or partial amnesia for the episode.

DOES IT EXIST?

Many investigators of this problem do not believe that pathological intoxication exists as an entity separable from other disorders. They argue that the unpredictable violent episodes represent dissociation states in which the alcohol drunk is incidental. Going berserk can happen to anyone under maximal stress whose ability to cope with enormous pressure has collapsed. Running amok and *negi negi** are acting-out syndromes in primitive societies that are related to the taboo of expressing strong personal feelings. They include impulsive, aimless destructiveness terminating in claims of amnesia. Even in the developed countries, unmotivated outbursts of hostile activities are becoming more common. Acute paranoid psychotic reactions are usually considered responsible for these aberrations. A number of patients with temporal lobe dysrhythmias manifest aggressiveness, hyperactivity, and deluded behavior. Genetic forms of sudden, unexpected violence are also described.

In recent years, abrupt, unthinking harm to one's self or others followed by an annestic episode has been caused by drugs other than ethanol. Phencyclidine toxicity can precisely duplicate what we understand as pathological intoxication. Acute amphetamine or cocaine psychosis is another condition that has to be considered. Barbiturates and similarly acting brain depressants are capable of inducing abrupt, assaultive outbursts. So a person who has taken a drink and had a rage reaction may have other important psychoactive drugs in his system.

Acute alcohol intoxication is known to be associated with purposeless violence, stuporousness, and amnesia (see Chapter 14, "Blackouts: 'You Mean I Did That Last Night?'"). But if the diagnosis of pathologic intoxication has any reason for existence as a discrete entity, it is in the hypersensitivity of a few people to modest, non-intoxicating amounts. Therefore, many unrelated behavioral disturbances have been misdiagnosed as pathological intoxication. This does not mean that the condition is non-existent. It means that it is not a frequent syndrome.

CRITERIA FOR THE DIAGNOSIS OF PATHOLOGICAL INTOXICATION

Although rather rare, instances of pathological intoxication do occur. It is neither difficult nor improper to make such a diagnosis under the following conditions.

---

*An atypical psychosis resembling latah found in Madagascar.

1. The person has either never used alcohol previously or has had a normal response to it in the past.

2. An insult to the brain, usually a substantial head injury or encephalitis, has taken place. Some students of the condition have suggested that pre-existing epilepsy; or unstable, hysterical personality; or cerebral arteriosclerosis may predispose to the pathological response to alcohol. Others have emphasized that severe levels of stress are of paramount importance in precipitating pathological intoxication. Even hypoglycemia has been suspected, but not proven, in a few cases. Perhaps the common denominator of all of the alleged contributory causes is impairment of cerebral nutrition or damage or death of specific inhibitory neurones.

3. Following recovery from the head trauma or other disorder, the person loses his tolerance to alcohol. He responds unthinkingly, impulsively, and belligerently to no or minor provocation after consuming alcohol. The amount may be as little as one or two ounces of ethanol. In order to make a secure diagnosis of pathological intoxication, a blood alcohol concentration of less than 0.1% seems necessary. Otherwise, pathological intoxication could not be differentiated from alcohol intoxication with an associated rage response.

4. A challenge with the same amount of alcohol reproduces the explosive behavior. It is preferable to give the drug intravenously so that the patient is unaware of when the alcohol is instilled. Sometimes attempts to reproduce the noxious behavior will not succeed in a neutral or benign environment. Whether the deliberate introduction of a stressor should be tried might be considered. Precautionary restraints may be indicated. A history of repeated, bizarre, spontaneous episodes following the moderate use of alcohol would favor the diagnosis.

5. Following the outburst (which may be brief or last for hours), a period of exhaustion and sleep intervenes. Upon awakening, the individual cannot remember the unusual events in which he was involved.

6. The offensive behavior should be atypical of the person's conduct when not drinking.

THE INTERACTION OF BRAIN DAMAGE AND ALCOHOL

It is well known that posttraumatic encephalopathy alone can be accompanied by unprovoked assaultiveness. A sudden burst of assaultive behavior following little or no provocation can be seen in those who have sustained cerebral damage from many causes, especially trauma.

High levels of alcohol intake are a major cause of criminal aggressive acts in this society. Drunkenness produces impaired judgment, reduction of controls over behavior, and paranoid misinterpretation of the environment. The result can be an alcohol-provoked rage.

Since both brain damage and alcohol themselves are capable of producing seriously aberrant behaviors, it is hardly surprising that the combination will do likewise. In the person who is susceptible to pathological intoxication, the brain damaged person requires the triggering action of small quantities of alcohol to unleash the hostility and its sequellae.

Pathological intoxication, therefore, exists as a narrow band on the continuum between the spontaneous violence of some brain damaged people and the overtly aggressive acts of those who lose control under the influence of large amounts of ethanol. Its existence is justified because these are people whose conduct disorders will be brought under control by complete abstinence from "social" amounts of beverage alcohol.

LOSS OF TOLERANCE TO ALCOHOL

Since pathological intoxication represents a serious loss of the ability to ingest alcohol, it may be useful to mention other circumstances in which tolerance to this substance is also diminished. People who have sustained previous head injuries may describe a loss of ability to "hold their liquor," even when the changes do not include hostile displays. Such individuals tend to pass out after a few drinks.

Usually, aging brings with it a diminution of tolerance. This is presumably due to a loss of the brain's ability to compensate for the psychomotor changes that accompany the intoxicated state. No doubt, the impaired metabolism of alcohol also contributes to their inability to deal with alcohol as well as they did during their younger years.

Naturally, people who stop sustained drinking practices will notice an increased sensitivity to lesser amounts when they resume drinking. It is generally believed that unusually fatigued persons or those with debilitating illnesses will be more affected by alcohol than was customary for them.

Liver damage severe enough to interfere with the enzyme systems that metabolize alcohol or acetaldehyde will cause blood and brain alcohol levels much higher than estimated in consideration of the quantity imbibed. End stage alcoholics without cirrhosis can lose some of their tolerance. This is ascribed to the diffuse brain damage resulting from chronic alcoholism.

FORENSIC ASPECTS

Criminal acts committed under circumstances in which pathological intoxication might be postulated represent an important defense of a person accused of an act of violence. The consumption of large amounts of alcohol might be a mitigating factor insofar as intent is concerned, when a major crime is executed. But if pathological intoxication can be proven, it may more readily constitute grounds for a verdict of involuntary manslaughter in a case of a homicide. This is especially true if the pathological violence is the first instance of such behavior. The defense may be invalidated if the defendant knows that he is prone to automatic violent deeds if he takes small amounts of alcohol.

The diagnosis of pathological intoxication is not easily made. A detailed case study must be done and the six criteria noted above substantially satisfied. One important differential diagnostic possibility must be excluded: malingering. Naturally, when the threat of punishment is anticipated, a lack of recall for the violent incident might be claimed. Inconsistencies in the story must be carefully sought. Polygraph tests, even the willingness to take such tests, may be helpful in forming a personal opinion, even if such testing is not admissible evidence in court.

DISCUSSION

The literature on pathological intoxication is quite confusing. A wide variety of bellicose disturbances that happen to occur in connection with drinking are randomly grouped together by some clinicians as pathological intoxication. These include psychomotor epilepsy, delirium tremens, violence resulting from drunkenness, and certain dissociation states.

Unfortunately, no reliable objective test is available to support the diagnosis. The recurrence of assaultive behavior under test conditions is supportive of the diagnosis when it occurs, but negative tests do not necessarily rule out the condition. Temporal lobe spiking on the electroencephalogram following the ingestion of small amounts of alcohol occurs only in a small percentage of these people.

Nevertheless, it is believed that this condition represents a rare but real diagnostic entity that can be sorted out from the other states mentioned. This opinion is held on the basis of clinical impressions of a small number of cases seen over the years that conformed to the criteria mentioned here.

The mechanism of the loss of tolerance to alcohol in pathological intoxication is worth investigating. Both tissue and behavioral intolerance may play a role. Tissue intolerance would result from the impaired neurones' being less able to withstand the toxic effect of alcohol. Behavioral loss of tolerance signifies that the adaptive and monitoring functions of the brain are diminished to the point that antisocial impulses cannot be controlled or modulated, and they come forth as impulsive, maladaptive behaviors.

BIBLIOGRAPHY

- Bach-Y-Rita, G., Lion, J. R. & Ervin, F. R. Pathological intoxication and electroencephalographic status. Amer. J. Psychiat. 127: 698–702, 1970.
- Coid, J. *Mania â potu:* A critical review of pathological intoxication. Psychological Med. 9: 709–719, 1979.
- Hollender, M. H. Pathological intoxication—Is there such an entity? J. Clin. Psychiat. 40: 424–426, 1979.
- Kosbab, F. P. and Kuhnley, E. J. Pathological intoxication. Psychiat. Opinion. 15: 35–38, 1978.
- Maletsky, B. M. The diagnosis of pathological intoxication. J. Studies Alcohol. 37: 1215–1228, 1976.

10. Alcohol and the Liver

New information is being generated concerning the metabolism of alcohol. This substance is a drug that seriously affects public health, any anything that is learned of its transformation in the body might be a help in treatment of acute and chronic alcohol toxicity.

Alcohol (also ethyl alcohol or ethanol) is quickly absorbed from the stomach and upper intestinal tract. Less than 10 percent is excreted unchanged from the lungs and skin and only a trace from the kidneys, so that the liver must deal with the bulk of ingested ethanol. Other organs do not have the necessary enzymes to metabolize it. So the liver cell is crucial in detoxifying alcohol and, as will be seen, impaired hepatic ability to metabolize alcohol causes further damage to the liver.

ALCOHOL, NUTRITION, AND LIVER DISEASE

At one time it was thought that a disease like cirrhosis was due to malnutrition rather than from the direct toxic effect of ethanol on the liver. After all, heavy drinkers spend little money for food and less time eating. Balanced diets are rarely consumed by alcoholics. Alcoholic gastritis causes a loss of appetite and vomiting if food is taken in. Alcoholic pancreatitis produces steatorrhea with its loss of nutriments.

Alcohol and its metabolites interfere with the release of water soluble vitamins from the liver. The metabolism of alcohol utilizes thiamine (vitamin B1), and alcoholic beverages contain hardly any vitamins. It is quite likely that a chronic heavy drinker will be malnourished in the essential vitamins and minerals.

This does not mean that he or she will be cachectic, although in the end stages of alcohol abuse that can certainly occur. Alcohol does have a caloric value of about 7 calories per gram, or about 1375 calories per pint of distilled spirts. This is more than half the daily caloric requirements for an average-sized person. A heavy imbiber of beer, wine, or whiskey may be obese but still could be malnourished in specific nutritional components such as vitamins, minerals, and proteins.

It is now well established that when chronic alcoholics do eat a balanced diet, they still may develop cirrhosis. Leiber and his associates fed a group of healthy volunteer subjects a very adequate diet plus vitamin and mineral supplements. They also received six drinks a day, or a total of 10 ounces of 86 proof alcohol daily for an 18-day period.

The investigators found a progressive rise in liver fat (by serial needle biopsies). At the end of the experiment there was eight times as much fat in the liver cells as at the start. The liver cells were distorted with striking changes in the mitochondria, the organelles, and the endoplasmic reticulum. During the 18-day period the blood alcohol concentration never rose above 90 mg/100 ml, which is below the level that is considered legally intoxicating.

These findings signify that consistent, spaced drinking, even without producing drunkenness, might still induce liver impairment over time. Cessation of drinking brought about a reversal of the fatty deposition in the liver.

These results were replicated in rats fed an adequate diet with 50 percent of their calories supplied as alcohol. The rats did not go on to develop alcoholic hepatitis or cirrhosis. Alcoholic cirrhosis is a later manifestation of liver toxicity (cirrhosis takes about 10 years to develop), and the rat's life span is only about 2 years. Lieber's group repeated their study on 16 longer-lived baboons, providing half the caloric requirement as alcohol and otherwise giving the animals an adequate diet. A control group received an alcohol-free diet of the same caloric content. The control group all had normal livers at the end of the study. The experimental group all turned out to have fatty livers, five baboons developed alcoholic hepatitis, and six others eventually showed cirrhorsis of the liver. No doubt the combination of large amounts of alcohol plus associated malnutrition induces cirrhosis more easily than either factor alone, but the experiments described above indicate that alcohol, by itself, is capable of causing cirrhosis.

THE METABOLISM OF ALCOHOL

The breakdown of alcohol in the liver proceeds over acetaldehyde to acetate, which eventually becomes water and carbon dioxide. This simple statement actually describes a complicated process involving a number of liver enzymes and coenzymes. The first step, the formation of acetaldehyde and hydrogen ions, is a significant one.

Ethyl alcohol	alcohol dehydrogenase	Acetaldehyde + Hydrogen ions
$CH_3 \cdot CH_2OH$		$CH_3 \cdot CHO + H_2$

The enzyme, alcohol dehydrogenase, is available to deal with the modest amount of alcohol produced by intestinal microorganisms acting on sugars. Alcohol manufactured in the intestine is almost entirely cleared in the liver before it can reach the systemic circulation.

The alcohol dehydrogenase pathway is rate limited. Other metabolic systems (catalase) can be brought into play when large amounts of alcohol are introduced into the organism. The auxiliary systems may account for the partial tolerance acquired by chronic drinkers.

The first breakdown product of alcohol metabolism, acetaldehyde, has a toxicity of its own. It impairs certain functions of the liver cell, which causes higher acetaldehyde levels in heavy drinkers than in non-alcoholics drinking similar amounts. High acetaldehyde levels disturb the synthesis of heart and skeletal muscle protein. In the brain acetaldehyde interferes with the metabolism of some of the neurotransmitters.

Hydrogen ions convert pyruvate, a step in the gluconeogenesis of protein to glucose, into lactate. If this happens when little or no carbohydrate is eaten, and when glycogen stores in the liver are depleted, hypoglycemia can result. A low blood sugar is a possible cause of the anxiety, shakiness, and mental confusion in some alcoholics. Prolonged, severe hypolglycemia could cause brain damage.

The excessive amounts of lactate diffuse into the blood stream and produce lactic acidosis. The kidneys cannot excrete uric acid well in the presence of lactic acidosis. Uric acid accumulates in the blood and other tissues producing hyperuricemia and gouty attacks. This explains the well-known association of gout with drinking bouts in predisposed individuals.

The excessive hydrogen ions derived from alcohol catabolism displace the hydrogen that would have been generated from the breakdown of fat. This means that lipids will accumulate and cause fatty infiltration of the liver. Even when no fat is ingested, a fatty liver can result from stored fat that is mobilized from body fat cells by alcohol-induced hormonal discharges from the liver, fat which the liver is incapable of handling.

The inability of the liver to metabolize fat produces a number of consequences. Some of the excess fat is combined into lipoproteins in the liver. The enzymes responsible for the reaction continue to be secreted even after alcohol has been eliminated, producing elevated lipoprotein levels in the blood. In predisposed people, alcohol acts to elevate their blood lipid level, with its danger of coronary atherosclerosis. Some of the excessive accumulation of fat is broken down to ketones. These are acid-reacting substances and, in combination with the lactic acidosis, can produce a ketoacidosis manifested by drowsiness, stupor, or coma.

The long-noted clinical observation that chronic alcoholics being detoxified are resistant to the effects of drugs like sedatives, tranquilizers, and anesthetic agents has been confirmed in the laboratory. The reason for the lack of effect of these drugs in ordinary doses is that alcohol induces excessive quantities of the enzymes that are also effective in metabolizing these other drugs. During active drinking, however, the alcohol interferes with the liver's ability to detoxify drugs and causes a prolongation of the drugs' effects and, perhaps, potentiation of the sedative effect of alcohol.

As liver cells become damaged from exposure to alcohol, their ability to degrade ethanol also fails. Serious hepatic insufficiency is one reason why heavy drinkers may lose their capacity to consume more than small amounts, because whatever alcohol is consumed continues to recycle. The well-known susceptibility of excessive drinkers to carbon tetrachloride poisoning might be explained on the basis of the competition of both drugs for certain hepatic enzymes.

Consistent drinking will cause fatty liver cells to become inflamed, with some cells becoming necrotic—alcoholic hepatitis. Still later, the inflammatory process causes scarification of the liver parenchyma—cirrhosis. The blood supply to many liver cells becomes impaired because of the scarring. The results of the partial or complete obstruction of the portal veins are many: esophageal and rectal varices with bleeding, ascites with worsening of the hypoproteinemia, uremia due to an inability to clear ammonia from the blood, and hepatic coma. In large urban areas cirrhosis is now the fourth leading cause of death in males between ages 25 and 45. Sudden deaths have occurred in people who had been drinking heavily enough to develop a very fatty liver. Fat emboli were found in the pulmonary vessels, and it is believed that the emboli came from the liver.

The synthesis of protein is impaired when the liver is damaged. This causes hypoalbuminemia with reversal of the albumin:globulin ratio. Prothrombin is not manufactured in sufficient quantities. Combined with a deficient intake of vitamin K, coagulation is defective, and hemorrhagic tendencies compound the danger when thin-walled varices rupture.

ALCOHOL AND SEXUAL DYSFUNCTIONS

The combination of impotence, gynecomastia, and testicular atrophy in male alcoholics was long assumed to be an effect of underlying liver damage. More recently it was found that the gynecomastia and atrophy of the testicles were seen in drinkers who had no evidence of substantial liver impairment.

Acute alcohol intake was shown to decrease the testicular synthesis and increase the metabolic disposition of testosterone. The decreased plasma testosterone levels lead to an increased leutinizing hormone production by a hypothalamic-pituitary feedback mechanism. These endocrine changes may explain the paradox noted by Shakespeare and many others that alcohol "provokes the desire but takes away the performance." Leutinizing hormone appears to increase sexual drive, but the low testosterone level does not permit sustained penile erection.

CIRRHOSIS AND CANCER OF THE LIVER

Primary cancer of the liver is not common in North America. Its substrate, in most cases, is cirrhosis. In Lee's series, only 11 percent of such malignancies occurred in nonalcoholic cirrhotics. In other parts of the world, cancer of the liver is often secondary to parasitic or viral liver disease. In this country, primary hepatic cancers develop at the site of hyperplastic liver nodules, which are regenerative attempts by the alcoholic's cirrhotic liver.

SUMMARY

In the absence of malnutrition large amounts of alcohol taken over extended periods of time can cause fatty liver, hepatitis, and, with continued drinking, progression to cirrhosis. It is difficult for a chronic alcoholic not to be malnourished in essential food elements so that these deficiencies contribute to the liver damage.

Excessive amounts of alcohol increase the synthesis of fat, prevent its breakdown, and mobilize peripheral fat. This results in fatty infiltration of the liver and elevated plasma lipoprotein levels with its consequences.

Heavy drinking can produce hypoglycemia by converting pyruvate, a precursor of glucose, to lactate. Contributory factors are a poor carbohydrate intake and a depleted glycogen reserve in the liver.

Hyperuricemia and gout can develop in predisposed individuals because of the lactic acidosis and its effect upon the renal tubule's ability to excrete uric acid.

Alcoholic ketoacidosis is due to a combination of increased ketones formed from the hyperlipemia and the shift in the Krebs cycle from pyruvate to lactate.

Large quantities of alcohol have dual effects on the metabolism of other drugs. Alcohol accelerates the metabolic breakdown of certain drugs, making the alcoholic being detoxified less sensitive to anesthetics, sedatives, and tranquilizers. The actively drinking alcoholic, however, may be more sensitive to such drugs because the metabolic pathways are preempted by alcohol.

The impotence of alcoholics is not necessarily caused by liver dysfunction, although it may be contributory. Rather, it may be a direct toxic effect upon gonadal steroid secretion.

Hyperplastic nodular cirrhosis is a favorable site for hepatoma development.

Acetaldehyde rather than alcohol may be the toxin involved in muscle, neuronal, and possibly hepatocyte dysfunction.

Hypoproteinemia, hypoprothrombinemia, hypovitaminosis, and their sequellae are a consequence of alcoholic liver disease.

BIBLIOGRAPHY

- *Alcohol and Health: New Knowledge*. Second Special Report to the Congress. Supt. of Documents, U.S. Govt. Printing Office, Washington, D.C., 20402, 1974.
- Kissen, B. and Begleiter, H. *The Biology of Alcoholism*. Plenum, New York, 1971–1973.
- Leiber, C. S. The metabolism of alcohol. *Scientific American*, 234:25–33, 1976.
- Leiber, C. S., et al. Sequential production of fatty liver, hepatitis and cirrhosis in subhuman primates fed with adequate diets. *Proc. Nat. Acad. Sci.*, 72:437–441, 1975.
- Lucia, S. P. Alcohol and the liver. *JAMA*, 229:391, 1974.

II

THE NATURE
OF ALCOHOLISM

11. How to Become an Alcoholic

With 10 percent of the drinking population having problems managing their drinking, it may seem superfluous to provide instructions on how to become an alcoholic. It apparently is an almost inevitable process for millions of our citizens. The point, of course, is that by learning of the techniques of drinking destructively, someone might use the information in order to avoid such practices. In this chapter, alcoholism is used to include both problem drinking and alcoholic addiction.

IN THE BEGINNING

A certain amount of the loading in favor of becoming alcoholic apparently happens when a certain sperm cell fertilizes a certain egg cell. The studies in which identical twins were raised either by their natural or adoptive parents indicate that inherited factors do have some impact upon subsequent drinking practices.

Identical twins, one raised by the natural alcoholic parents and one by adoptive, non-alcoholic parents, will have similar rates of alcohol-related disorders. When an identical twin of non-alcoholic parents is raised by alcoholic adoptive parents—one or both—the chances of that twin becoming alcoholic is approximately the same as the twin raised by the biologic parents.

How strong are these factors in determining whether a child will become an alcoholic? Not very great. Although one or both parents may have been considered to be alcoholics, neither may have possessed the genetic predisposition. Even if a child has inherited the genetic component, it amounts to no more than a vulnerability to become an alcoholic. Therefore, children of families with numbers of inordinate drinkers have a responsibility to themselves to be particularly careful about using alcoholic beverages. Whether it is, indeed, a genetically determined effect in any specific child is unknown. It is just as likely to be an acquired family tradition to drink excessively. In both instances dangerous drinking practices can be avoided by being aware of the vulnerability. To slip into the family's pattern has only one advantage. One can always blame it on one's chromosomes.

THE MILIEU

Much more important than heredity are the environmental impacts—the strong conditioning one acquires from relatives, friends, peer groups, media, educators, pastors, and others about how to deal with life stress, and how to drink.

It is possible for some young people to wind up as adult alcoholics by being either neglected or overprotected during their early growing-up period. Neglect deprives the child of suitable role models to emulate. Learning how to relate to other people, a process that should begin within the family group, takes place elsewhere or not at all. Non-caring parents surrender the training of the youngster to anyone or any group that happens to be in contact with the child rather than to a devoted family unit. Neglect deprives the child of needed supports in time of crisis.

Overprotection is equally detrimental. Independence, self-esteem, and problem-solving and decision-making abilities are not acquired. The maturational process atrophies. The child's ability to endure difficult experiences, loss, frustration, and defeat remains undeveloped. In other words, the immaturity imposed upon the young person helps to shape alcohol-consuming behavior and, in fact, many other undesirable adult behaviors.

We are not sure of what an ideal upbringing consists of, but certain features of the parent-child interaction like love, trust, consistency, concern (not over-concern), willingness to permit the child to assume responsibilities, and a relationship that permits the discussion of problems are certainly components of a helpful atmosphere in which to grow up.

ON BECOMING AN ALCOHOLIC

One way to get into trouble with drinking is being able to hold your liquor better than most people. Unfortunately, folk knowledge assumes the opposite. But being able to consume unusually large quantities before becoming affected by it simply means that the body is exposed to and must deal with the inordinate amounts being poured in. The ability to remain relatively sober while others slide under the table unable to drink more may be due either to the development of tolerance after consistent exposure to ethanol, being a very large person (because alcohol diffuses uniformly into all cells), or having some metabolic facility in dealing with the chemical.

Regarding resistance to the intoxicating affects of liquor, a vivid description of Jack London's ability to handle alcoholic beverages can be found in his memoirs "John Barleycorn."* London died at age 40, a suicide with advanced alcoholic hepatitis and nephritis. As a child, he discovered his amazing ability to drink long and hard without passing out. He never liked the taste of booze, but drunkenness was the social norm on the San Francisco Bay waterfront of the day, and he worked hard achieving a rousing intoxication whenever his friends and the bars were available.

But there are many other ways to become an alcoholic, and some of them should be mentioned. Denial and rationalization are two psychological techniques used to avoid the reality of impending or existing trouble with one's drinking. Although the consequences of drinking are disastrous—job losses, arrests, family problems, car accidents, and so forth—these are often considered reasons to drink rather than reasons to terminate one's drinking. This sort of evasion of the reality situation is a common way to become a confirmed alcoholic.

Certain health problems are alcohol related. Specific kinds of liver damage, pancreatitis, gastritis, and in the later stages, neuritis, esophageal varicosities, and other ailments are evidence that the body is not successfully handling the amount of alcohol imbibed. Obviously, a decision has to be made about drinking, but all too often it is either abrogated or the physical distress itself becomes a reason to drink more.

Many people drink because of unease, anxiety, and depression. For example, "drowning one's sorrows" is an everyday expression. Alcohol may erase these noxious feelings, but it is well documented that as one continues to imbibe, tension and anxiety levels rise again. Furthermore, the morning-after state is often quite unpleasant. Therefore, something is needed to ease the psychological and physical unpleasantness. Alcohol reverses the miserable feelings, but it may produce an endless cycle of dysphoria → drinking → dysphoria → drinking.

The positive rewards of moderate drinking are not to be ignored since they involve 90 percent of all users of beverage alcohol, the non-problem drinkers. Tension relaxation, a smoothing-out of interpersonal irritants, perhaps a distancing from the immediacy of life's travails are some of the positive reinforcers of small amounts of ethanol.

Repeated loss of control over drinking, however, is an ominous sign for the consumer. Successful social drinkers use certain cues that tell them when to stop. It may be a matter of counting the number of drinks or drinking only during specific social occasions. Maintenance of control may also be managed either by an internal feedback mechanism that estimates how high one feels or by

---

*John Barleycorn: Alcoholic Memoirs by Jack London. Reprinted by Robert Bentley, Cambridge, Mass. 02139, 1964.

whether any signs of incoordination or slurring of speech are perceptible. These become stop signals for the modest drinker. People who are unaware of or who deliberately ignore these internal or external warning cues are at risk of over-drinking even when they have no intention of doing so.

Counseling certain alcoholics includes teaching the stop signals and teaching how to respond to them. A few chronic alcoholics demonstrate another sort of loss of control. A single drink precipitates a drinking spree. They appear unable to stop once primed by a small amount of alcohol. People with problems of loss of control must either abstain completely, learn strategies of maintaining control, or accept inevitable alcoholism.

Mental attitudes toward the symbolic meaning of drinking may trap some people into a career of excessive consumption, culminating in alcoholism. The notion that drinking a lot is macho, or that, as in the case of young people, being intoxicated is manly, can lead to precarious drinking patterns. Naturally, this sort of symbolism is used in media advertising extensively. One can hardly watch television, listen to the radio, or read newspapers or magazines without acquiring the feeling that drinking is either a prestigious, a manly (or womanly) conduct, the equivalent of friendship and camaraderie, the high road to the good life, virility or any of the other positive values.

In between the commercials, the entertainment content does nothing to dispute these claims. In fact, it reinforces them. It seems that cinema directors have settled on the idea that the only way to project strong emotions involving severe pressure or desperate decision making on the screen is to have the actor gulp drinks. A 1-gulp scene appears to be equated to lesser pressures such as a rough day at work, but a 4- or 5-gulper means serious trouble. A recent television film showed the male lead downing shot after shot of what must have been strong tea because obvious signs of intoxication did not appear. This and a stern face was how he portrayed how desperate things were with him. Does such permeating propaganda cause or contribute to eventual alcoholism in some people?

Preoccupation with drink and securing one's supply lines are evidence of psychological dependence. The stash may be placed in the gastrointestinal tract in anticipation of an evening when potable beverages will not be provided. It may be in the car, on the person, or concealed around the house or garden, just in case the normal availability of alcohol is threatened, as it is on Election Day.

THE MANY ROADS TO ALCOHOLISM

There are many mental attitudes that help produce a problem drinker or an alcohol addict. The following list provides some of the proven approaches to achieving the status of being an alcoholic. These should be considered danger signals.

• Ignore the need for morning drinks to control tremulousness as being anything of consequence.

• Pay no attention to the fact that you have blacked out during a drinking bout or two.

• Having had the DTs means that you were, by definition, addicted to alcohol. Not doing anything about it perpetuates the situation.

• Do not listen to anyone—family, friend, or doctor—who advises you to stop or markedly cut down on your drinking.

• If you do decide to stop or cut back and find you can't—well, you tried.

• If you have had a series of accidents while drunk, don't worry about it. You only drink as much as the other guys.

• If you find you're losing your ability to drink without getting drunk, it's not important.

• Your father and grandfather were drunks, so what's the use of fighting it?

• If it weren't for booze, you'd be a nervous wreck.

• There's nothing wrong with persistent thinking of the next drink, giving drinking high priority, and assuring that your supplies are sufficient to take care of dry spells.

• You can't be an alcoholic. You only go on binges for a couple of weeks—two or three times a year.

SUMMARY

The drinking of the alcoholic differs in a number of ways from the drinking of a person who has no problems with the drug and who is not addicted to it. The wide diversity of alcoholic persons makes universal statements difficult, but certain behaviors that foster unsafe drinking are present with fair regularity in alcoholics.

The alcoholic seems to depend on alcohol as an exclusive technique of dealing with stress, boredom, and other unpleasant emotional states. The alcoholic has difficulty being realistic about his use of alcohol. The fact that he drank modestly for years and that now his intake has increased drastically is ignored or rationalized. Alcohol becomes a dominant and, eventually, an exclusive theme of one's existence. The stimulus-response aspect of drinking generalizes so that while, at one time, drinking was restricted to certain situations, eventually, it becomes a response to all situations. Some of the difficulties of treating the alcoholic person arise from these differences.

12. Alcohol-Related Disorders: Early Identification

Many aspects of the 1980 presidential race were unusual, but in one respect it was unique. Never before have four of the leading candidates or would-be candidates had close relatives who have publicly acknowledged that they had been in trouble with alcohol.

Betty Ford, Billy Carter, Joy Baker and Joan Kennedy made frank statements about their drinking problems and their treatment experiences. Many other prominent politicians, executives, sports figures, and entertainers have recently come forth and announced similar difficulties.

It is heartening to see that the symbolic closet where alcoholics have traditionally secluded themselves is now open and that those in need of help are seeking it at an earlier phase of their drinking careers. Healthy cultural shifts appear to be underway that will provide an opportunity for the earlier diagnosis and treatment of problem drinkers.

Health professionals must prepare themselves for the new situation, sharpening their diagnostic skills, detecting early dysfunctional drinking, and developing effective techniques for motivating and managing the pre-alcoholic. In an effort to detect the premonitory signs and symptoms of dysfunctional drinking, a review of the danger signals is attempted here. In general, these are signals, not diagnostic certainties. They are intended to arouse suspicion that the patient may be at risk of impairing himself or herself if drinking continues at the current level. The signals to be mentioned are medical indicators. Very often behavioral and interpersonal danger signs coexist (see Chapter 11, "How to Become an Alcoholic," and Chapter 22, "How Social Drinkers Become Alcoholics").

THE "HITTING BOTTOM" NOTION

Many individuals and groups, including AA, have espoused the belief that before a drinker can really be driven to begin the recovery process he must "hit bottom." This means that his health must be severely impaired, his family situation wrecked, his finances depleted, or his self-respect shattered. Only then can he mobilize sufficient willpower to start the long, hard road back to sobriety and rehabilitation. Short of "hitting bottom," rationalizations that he can stop drinking whenever he wants to or that his misfortunes are not really due to excessive drinking may persist.

For some, it may be necessary to be confronted with a total personal disaster before sufficient resolve finally to stop using alcohol is achieved. On the other hand, this critical point may occur too late. By then, brain damage may be irreparable, liver failure irreversible, or the social situation may be irretrievable.

Therefore, our present efforts should be directed at early case finding and entry into treatment during mid-level drinking careers rather than during the final stages. Mid-level drinking disorders are more difficult to identify and are at a phase when it is harder to persuade the patient of the need to make major changes in his life. The conventional treatment methods may not be appropriate for these incipient alcoholics, and improved or alternative measures may have to be employed.

ALCOHOL-RELATED DISEASES OR SYMPTOMS

A sizable number of disorders are directly or indirectly associated with injudicious alcohol consumption. These abnormalities are not invariably associated with alcohol, but their presence should raise the possibility of that etiology. Furthermore, like intoxication or hangover, the frequency—not the existence—of these events will determine the degree of risk of impending alcoholism.

Alcoholic Fatty Liver, Pancreatitis, and Gastritis

A smooth non-tender enlargement of the liver with or without abnormal liver function tests in connection with drinking episodes is evidence of higher levels of ethanol intake than the liver cells can successfully metabolize. Severe, constant upper abdominal pain and tenderness usually radiating to the back reflects pancreatic inflammation and that too many years of excessive drinking already have occurred. Anorexia, nausea, and sometimes-bloody vomiting, is evidence of a direct toxic effect of alcohol on the stomach lining with associated erosions or ulcerations.

Poor Nutrition and Immune Response

In addition to an inattention to proper nutrition and hygienic measures, a preoccupation with drinking will cause a variety of pulmonary infections from aspiration while drunk to a failure of the normal pulmonary defense mechanisms.

Impaired absorption of nutrients and vitamins, particularly thiamine, and changes in intestinal motility contribute to the diarrhea that sometimes accompanies drinking bouts. Many other nutritional deficiencies can be identified.

Neurologic Changes

An increased patellar reflex has been noted in alcohol abusers. The earliest signs of peripheral neuropathy would include somewhat diminished touch, temperature, pain, and position sensations. Atrophy of the calf muscles early in the course of excessive drinking has been described by a few authors.

Hematologic Abnormalities

A number of hematologic changes can be caused by a variety of alcohol-related disturbances. These include a folate deficiency producing megaloblastosis or macrocytosis detectable in an elevated mean corpuscular volume. Pyridoxine deficiency can result in a sideroblastic anemia. Obscure instances of thrombocytopenia and bleeding may be traced to alcohol overuse.

Myopathy

Lower extremity muscle aches, weakness, cramping, and tenderness may be symptoms of alcoholic myopathy, and these can occur rather early in the evolution of the drinking career. Cardiomyopathy, on the other hand, is a late evidence of alcoholism.

The Skin and Alcohol

Long before rhinophyma, acne rosacea, and spider nevi make their appearance, less obvious alterations of the skin become noticeable. The face may be puffy, the cheeks and nose flushed, and the conjunctival vessels injected. The tongue is smooth and red (except when it is coated with chlorophyll), reflecting a vitamin B deficiency. Palmar erythema may be visible before cirrhosis can be diagnosed.

Cigarette burns between the index and middle fingers or on the chest, and contusions and bruises should be considered suspicious of alcoholic stupor and injury. Insect bites and frostbites are some of the hazards of spending a night out-of-doors in an alcoholic coma.

Blackouts

Loss of recall for a period of time when the drinker was apparently conscious and functioning well is not always a tardive sign of alcoholism. Amnesia for the hours or days of a drinking bout may occur shortly after heavy drinking has commenced and tend to recur during subsequent sprees.

Impotence and Loss of Libido

Male impotence can be an acute or a chronic consequence of considerable drinking. Alcohol appears to block the synthesis of testosterone in the gonads while accelerating its breakdown in the liver. Libido decrease is a somewhat later symptom resulting from low levels of testosterone availability or from its conversion to estrogen-like substances.

Cancer and Alcohol

Drinking alcoholic beverages leads to an increased risk of cancer at various sites of the body. Heavy drinking is associated with an increased probability of developing cancers of the tongue, mouth, pharynx, larynx, esophagus, and liver. Heavy alcohol and tobacco use act synergistically to increase the rate of head and neck cancers. Although alcohol is not a carcinogen, it may either act as a co-carcinogen or as a solvent for cancer-producing polyaromatic hydrocarbons.

LABORATORY AIDS IN THE DIAGNOSIS OF IMPENDING ALCOHOLISM

The demonstration of a positive blood alcohol and blood acetaldehyde during or shortly after drinking is not a valuable prognostic indicator of impending alcoholism. One possible exception is elevated blood alcohol levels associated with fairly normal behavior. It might indicate high levels of tolerance.

An elevated blood lactate simply reflects the shift from pyruvate to lactate metabolism. Lactic acidosis, however, decreases uric acid excretion and results in hyperuricemia or even attacks of gout. These latter findings are suspicious but not confirmatory of excessive use of ethanol.

Selective individuals may show a rise in serum triglycerides shortly after alcohol use. Such elevations return to normal within two weeks of abstinence. The very-low-density lipoproteins and chylomicrons are elevated and may remain high if alcohol is used chronically. When severe liver damage supervenes, plasma lipid levels will fall below normal because of an inability of the liver to synthesize lipoproteins.

Alcoholic acidosis and ketosis in the absence of diabetes, especially if accompanied by urinary ketone bodies, are suggestive of recent, heavy, binge-type drinking.

A very low blood sugar in a heavy drinker suggests that glycogen stores are exhausted, and alcohol metabolism is preventing gluconeogenesis from fat and amino acids. Since hypoglycemia has many causes, it is not diagnostic of alcohol excess, but it should always be considered in instances of coma in someone with alcohol on his breath.

Serum gamma-glutamyl transpeptidase (GGT) is elevated in drinkers who may have little evidence of hepatic malfunction. Although it gradually decreases during the abstinent period, it may remain elevated for weeks after cessation of heavy drinking. It may serve as a useful screening test for patients entering a medical care unit for reasons other than an alcohol problem. It is not completely specific for alcoholic liver dysfunction. An elevated GGT in the absence of barbiturate use or bilary disease is good supportive evidence for dysfunctional drinking and should be so considered by the physician and the patient.

Serum glutamic oxalacetic transaminase (SGOT), serum glutamic pyruvic transaminase (SGPT), lactic dehydrogenase (LDH), and similar enzymatic tests are all non-specific in that they are elevated in response to muscle injury, use of certain drugs, acute liver and kidney damage, etc. The GGT is fairly specific for liver damage or barbiturate use. It is, perhaps, most useful for alcoholic liver impairment, remaining elevated after the other enzyme tests have reverted to normal.

Low folic acid, thiamine, and phosphate levels have been reported in abstinent alcoholic patients, and these might be considered supportive of a diagnosis of excessive drinking.

Efforts to develop empirical markers of alcoholism—for example, the alpha-aminobutyric acid:leucine ratio—have not yet been refined to the point where they are clinically feasible.

In a recent article, Morse and Hurt summarize their use of laboratory findings in alcohol problems. They consider a patient to be an alcoholic if he comes in for a general examination with a blood alcohol level (BAL) of more than 100 mg/dl, if the BAL is 150 mg/dl without signs of intoxication, or if a BAL of 300 mg/dl is obtained at any time. Sixty-three percent of patients admitted to the alcoholism unit at Mayo Clinic had an elevated GGT. The SGOT was abnormal in 48 percent, and macrocytosis as measured by the mean corpuscular volume was abnormal in 26 percent. Serum triglycerides were elevated in 22 percent, alkaline phosphotase in 16 percent, serum bilirubin in 13 percent, and serum uric acid in 10 percent.

A recent development has been the combined use of the SMA12, the SMA6, and the complete blood count as a method for establishing a diagnosis of early alcoholism. These tests are routinely requested and do not add to patient costs. Utilizing this battery of 25 tests and applying a quadratic discriminant analysis to the data, Ryback et al. were able to predict 94 percent of alcoholics in treatment programs and 100 percent of non-alcoholics correctly. Sixteen of 23 alleged non-alcoholics who drank more than 3 drinks a day were also found to give positive results. The test was not accurate for those over 65 years of age. When the statistical software for the test becomes available, it may become a valuable screening device in physician's offices and hospital admission services.

SUMMARY

Assuredly, many patients with suspicious physical or laboratory evidence of incipient alcoholism will refuse to act on this information. Nevertheless, they should be informed of their situation as they would be in the early stages of any illness that is detected.

Some patients will take appropriate corrective action on their own or with the assistance of a therapist. Early identification and intervention is possible and, with skilled treatment, will be more rewarding than caring for chronic, end stage alcoholics.

BIBLIOGRAPHY

- Morse, R.M. and Hurt, R. D. Screening for alcoholism. JAMA 242:2688–2690, 1979.
- Ryback, R. S., Eckardt, M. J. and Pautler, C. P. Bio-chemical and hematological correlates of alcoholism. Research Communications in Chemical Pathology and Pharmacology, in press.

13. Hangover

Hangovers, a source of misery for those who have them and of amusement for those nearby, rarely require medical attention. Nevertheless, they provide an interesting component of the varieties of alcohol experiences.

The causes and consequences of the hungover state following immoderate alcohol consumption have not been completely clarified. Although it is a frequent event, the hangover has, until recently, not been as thoroughly studied as some of the other alcohol-related conditions. It is a self-limited disorder, and despite the appreciable distress involved, it is ordinarily treated with folk remedies. Much of the current research on this postintoxication state comes from Finland, where it is recognized as a considerable cause of absenteeism and decreased productivity.

SYMPTOMS AND SIGNS

This unpleasant interlude, following acute alcohol intoxication by 8 to 12 hours, has a long list of manifestations. Perhaps the most frequently encountered is a splitting headache, made worse by movement, bright lights, and loud sounds. Upper gastrointestinal symptoms of heartburn, loss of appetite, nausea, and vomiting are frequent. Dry mouth and a severe thirst are annoying and common. Nystagmus can be observed, and interestingly enough, it is opposite in direction to the to and fro movements of the eye seen during the acute intoxicated state: if the quick component of the movement is to the left during intoxication, it will be to the right during the hangover.

In addition to the headache, other central nervous system and autonomic system side effects include dizziness, sweating, tremulousness, pallor, palpitations, and sometimes insomnia. During this period, anxiety, depression, or both may be noted. Generalized symptoms of malaise and tiredness are frequent complaints.

CAUSES AND CONSEQUENCES

This array of symptoms and signs can hardly result from some single cause. The present idea about the etiology of the hangover is that a number of contributing factors combine to produce the picture with certain factors being dominant in specific instances. Needless to say, what is presented here should be seen as an interim explanation of the postalcoholic syndrome.

The Stress Response

Acute alcoholic intoxication is a physiologically stressful condition, made worse by associated factors such as lack of sleep, heavy smoking, and various feelings evoked by one's uninhibited behavior. A non-specific adrenergic response can be measured that precipitates a release of ACTH and cortisol and, perhaps, increased hypothalamic dopaminergic activity leading to a secondary inhibition of dopamine release. Moreover, elevated free fatty acid and triglyceride levels correlate quite well with the severity of hangover. These are changes that are expected following a stress reaction. Plasma testosterone levels are also known to be depressed during stress, and they are found to be lower during the postintoxication state.

Whether these endocrine shifts produce actual symptoms of hangover is not known, but they may contribute to their severity.

Hypoglycemia

Many of the manifestations of the hangover are reminiscent of hypoglycemia. Ethanol is known to lower blood glucose concentrations in the fasting state. In addition, not eating and vomiting add to the reduction of available carbohydrates. The blood glucose levels are at their lowest at the height of the hangover, but no differences in glucose concentrations are detectable between the mild and the severe hangovers. Therefore, in itself, hypoglycemia may worsen the postintoxication syndrome, but is only infrequently a primary cause of the state.

Acidosis

It is well established that ethanol produces a metabolic—and occasionally a respiratory—acidosis. The pH of the blood falls significantly during the hangover phase, at the same time that blood lactate and total ketone bodies are rising. The accumulation of organic acids and ketones resulting from the degradation of ethanol in the liver accounts for the ketoacidosis. The degree of acidosis correlates fairly well with the hangover's intensity and may be at least partially involved in its genesis. Fructose, a sugar currently in favor for the treatment of hangover, will reduce ketone body concentrations and also return blood pH and glucose levels to normal. But in controlled studies fructose had no measurable effect on the intensity either of the acute intoxicated state or of the postintoxicated state.

Acetaldehyde

Some of the effects of the postintoxication syndrome resemble the alcohol-Antabuse reaction, which is manifested by high acetaldehyde levels. Therefore, it is natural to look at acetaldehyde as a possible cause. It was found that the blood acetaldehyde curve was similar to the ethanol curve, so that all the acetaldehyde had been eliminated before the hangover began. Thus, acetaldehyde hardly can be a major etiologic factor in hangover induction.

Dehydration and Hyperhydration

A good candidate for a supporting role in the pathogenesis of hangovers is water balance alterations. It has been amply confirmed that alcohol intake first decreases and then increases the secretion of vasopressin, the antidiuretic hormone, from the posterior pituitary gland. This leads to a retention and later a diuresis of urine. Although much fluid may be ingested during a drinking bout, more will be voided. The increased urinary excretion can lead to dehydration. In addition, water loss during sweating, vomiting, and diarrhea will add to the fluid depletion, symptomatically manifested as dry mouth and thirst. On the other hand, as blood alcohol levels drop, antidiuretic hormone is stimulated, and hyperhydration can develop during the hangover.

Congeners

The congeners (fusel oil) are organic alcohols and salts formed when alcoholic beverages are manufactured. They include methanol, propanol, butyl and amyl alcohol, ethyl acetate, and ethyl formate. Vodkas, which are essentially diluted alcohol, contain the least, and bourbons and brandies contain the most fusel oil. Congeners provide the flavor and aroma of the beverage.

Congeners have been suspected of hangover production for some time. But they are present in only small amounts and can hardly play an important role. Furthermore, pure ethanol has been amply shown to induce the hungover state. At most, fusel oil can only contribute to the condition by competing with ethyl alcohol for its metabolizing enzyme, alcohol dehydrogenase.

Local Toxic Effects of Alcohol

The gastrointestinal upset, a prominent hangover feature, may be directly produced by alcohol, especially in its more concentrated forms. Alcohol stimulates the secretion of hydrochloric acid, and is known to produce inflammatory and erosive changes of the stomach lining. The nausea and vomiting may be a result of an acute gastritis that follows one or more heavy encounters with ethanol.

Alcohol

It appears that a necessary, but not a sufficient, condition for causing a hangover is a large enough quantity of alcohol. Some heavy drinkers, though, claim never to have had one, and other consumers complain of distressing "morning after" disturbances following rather moderate imbibing. Some of this variance may be related to psychological factors. It has been found that those drinkers who have negative attitudes toward drinking have more severe hangover symptoms than those with positive attitudes toward their drinking.

Although it is generally believed that the amount consumed relates to the appearance and severity of the hangover, no study could be found to prove the point. As indicated, the hangover probably has a multifactorial etiology with alcohol being the major element involved.

The central role of alcohol in the development of hangovers is underlined by a number of alcohologists who believe that the postintoxication syndrome is a manifestation of early withdrawal. Even after a single drinking bout a certain degree of tolerance develops. As evidence to support this point of view they mention that, at similar blood alcohol concentrations (BAC), symptoms of intoxication are less on the descending limb of the BAC than they were on the ascending limb. Hangover symptoms are viewed as rebound effects of early withdrawal. The fact that resuming drinking will reverse the symptomatology is cited as additional evidence for the concept.

TREATMENT

The "hair of the dog that bit you" treatment of the hangover is a traditional one. This use of a small amount of alcohol to correct the metabolic rebound is justifiable if it does not lead to another round of overdrinking. It is also rational if we accept the early withdrawal concept of the hangover.

To correct the acidosis, water balance disturbance, and low blood sugar, fluids such as orange juice would seem indicated. Rest and time will correct the other changes induced by the overindulgence. There is no objection to mild analgesics for the hangover headache. Sedatives and tranquilizers are not indicated.

SUMMARY

It would be interesting to know whether anyone has ever stopped drinking because of one or more severe hangovers. If so, then hangovers may have a protective quality for some people. On the other hand, their punishing psycho-physical effects may serve to reinforce a dysfunctional drinking pattern since relief is obtained by returning to alcohol.

The causes of the hangover are multiple, but alcohol is a necessary element. Other factors intervene to determine the nature and extent of the symptoms. The notion that we are dealing with an early alcohol withdrawal syndrome is worth exploring further.

BIBLIOGRAPHY

- Anylian, G. H., Dorn, J. and Swerdlow, J. The manifestations and assessment of ethanol-induced hangover. South African Med. J. 54:193, 1978.
- Linkola, J., Fykrquist, F. and Ylikahri, R. H. Renin, aldosterone and cortisol during ethanol intoxication and hangover. Acta Physiol. Scand. 106:75, 1979.
- Ylikahri, R. H. and Huttunen, M. U. Metabolic and endocrine pathology during hangover. In: *Alcohol Intoxication and Withdrawal IIIb*, Ed.: M. M. Gross, Plenum, N.Y., 1977.

14. Blackouts: "You Mean I Did That Last Night?"

The amnesia (blackout) that follows the drinking of large amounts of alcoholic beverages is an important medical and legal matter. Blackouts can be defined as the inability to remember a part or all of a drinking episode, even though consciousness was neither significantly clouded nor lost.

An alcoholic grayout is an intoxicated state after which recent prior events can be recalled only with difficulty. Passing out consists of becoming stuporous or comatose in connection with drinking and, therefore, having no memory for anything that may have happened.

PHENOMENOLOGY

Blackouts can occur in both nonalcoholics and alcoholics who have drunk a good deal. In fact, Jellinek and others have considered these acute anterograde amnesias to be a prodromal sign of chronic alcoholism. Jellinek's triad of early alcohol addiction consisted of blackouts, benders, and loss of control, with blackouts usually appearing before the other two manifestations.

Predisposing factors include gulping drinks and not eating, suggesting that it is a rapid rise in the blood alcohol concentration that induces the amnesia. However, a blackout may become evident only after the first few days of binge drinking. Lack of sleep plays a role in its induction. Those who have sustained a blackout are likely to have subsequent ones. Some people report that they experienced them on every episode of heavy drinking. Other heavy drinkers never seem to have blackouts. The highest incidence of blackouts occurs in those heavy drinkers who have considerable craving, who have a tolerance to alcohol, and who are solitary, gulping drinkers. In Tarter and Sugerman's series, loss of control, head trauma, and whiskey drinking were found to be positive factors. A family history of blackouts was not correlated with the condition. This group of alcoholic patients was separated into cravers and noncravers of alcohol. Blackouts were reported by the cravers as follows: never, 15.5 percent; sometimes, 48.3 percent; often, 22.4 percent; and almost every time, 13.8 percent. The noncravers had fewer blackouts, with 35.3 percent saying that they never had them, 58.8 percent saying that they sometimes had them, and the remaining 5.9 percent reporting that they had them almost every time.

The amnesic intervals can last for days or for shorter blocks of time. They are not restricted to certain significant events; instead they consist of a complete memory loss for everything that happened. Neither the person involved nor those around him are ordinarily aware of the memory defect. He may go through the motions of functioning adequately, and may not even seem very intoxicated to others.

Meanwhile, the blood alcohol level will be between 150 and 300 mg/dl. Generally, the drinker will awaken after sleeping it off and be unable to remember what happened the evening before. If the events are related to him in detail, he still will not be able to recall them. If nothing of note happened and witnesses do not try to remind him, he may not be aware that a blackout occurred.

During the state, a person functions more or less adequately, conversing, driving, and performing other well-learned acts. Someone may start drinking in Los Angeles and awaken in a hotel room in St. Louis a few days later quite unable to remember how he arrived there or anything that happened during the period.

Such profound memorial deficits can be accounted for by an inability to transfer short-term memories to long-term storage sites. The person is able to continue to perform because immediate memory (up to a minute) is retained, and the retrieval of information from the long-term memory banks is only partially disturbed. It is the transfer process of short-term data (what happened more than a minute ago) to the permanent memory stores that is knocked out. Thus, a memory gap exists, and it cannot be filled in by cueing the person or by attempting to retrieve the missing information under hypnosis or sodium pentothal.

It is entirely possible that alcoholic blackouts are much more common than we assume. A brief memory gap lasting minutes may not come to awareness, and even long ones may be ignored.

A lesser condition that could be called cocktail party transient and partial amnesia becomes observable when the drinker later tries to remember the contents of what seemed to be a significant conversation at the time. Memory losses occur in nonalcoholic drinkers after considerably lower doses than those associated with the blackout. A decreased ability to recall may take place at blood alcohol levels of 40 mg/dl, and it progresses in a linear fashion as the level rises.

CAUSATION

We can say what blackouts are not, even though we do not know what causes them. They are not the psychological repression of traumatic, "forgotten" incidents. They are usually not instances of state-dependent learning since recall for the amnesic period will not take place during subsequent intoxications. They are not produced by structural alterations in the brain, since they are readily reversible, and tests of short-term memory function under sober conditions are within normal limits. Hypoglycemia has been ruled out as a causative factor.

Alcohol is one of the few substances known that induces substantial memory gaps in the presence of a consciousness that is relatively unimpaired. Puromycin, an antineoplastic and antitrypanosomal antibiotic, has also been shown to impair the storage of data into the memory banks, apparently by interfering with the metabolism of protein—specifically of RNA. The metabolism of the processing of new information and of its storage is probably disturbed when sufficient concentrations of alcohol are in contact with brain cells involved in the transfer.

An interesting speculation deals with the relationship of blackouts, presumably a toxic process, to the amnestic-confabulatory syndrome of Wernicke-Korsakoff. The latter is an organic condition, usually caused in this country by chronic heavy drinking and more precisely by the thiamine deficiency that accompanies alcoholism. Degenerative changes in the diencephalon, particularly the hippocampus, are seen at autopsy. It is possible that a patient with repeated blackouts eventually goes on to develop the Wernicke-Korsakoff array of symptoms. If so, is it possible that high-dose vitamin B therapy may prevent or attenuate blackouts?

It might be assumed that those who sustain a complete loss of memory for hours or days would be sufficiently frightened to discontinue using the substance that caused the deficit. Unfortunately, blackouts only infrequently result in abstinence. Individuals who experience multiple amnesias seem to accept them as the price one pays for intoxication, and they equate them with the memory loss that accompanies passing out. These are completely different conditions. Passing out is associated with the inability to function actively. During a blackout, a person can still perform, appear normal, and as we shall see, become a hazard to himself and others.

DIFFERENTIAL DIAGNOSIS

Not everyone who experiences a memory loss during alcohol intoxication has a blackout. Any disruption of the hippocampal complex can evoke an amnestic response. The Wernicke-Korsakoff syndrome has been mentioned. Certain head traumas (the postconcussion syndrome) or hypoxia of the brain (as in carbon monoxide poisoning) may sometimes present a similar picture.

Simulating amnesia by malingering in order to try to evade responsibility for some act must be considered. The amnesias that accompany deliria or coma are readily differentiated because of the profound alterations of consciousness. Psychogenic amnesias occur preponderantly during war or natural disasters as a part of a severe stress syndrome. They may also take place during catastrophic events involving one or a small number of people. Memories blacked out by severe stress are often retrievable under dissociating agents like hypnosis or sodium pentothal, differentiating them from blackouts.

LEGAL SIGNIFICANCE

Blackouts assume a legal importance when some major accident or crime has occurred, and the accused was intoxicated at the time of the incident. The individual may disclaim any knowledge of the accident, assault, or homicide and of the events leading up and subsequent to it. Questions to be posed to expert witnesses are whether such a person is capable of premeditating a crime and whether the capacity to understand the nature of the criminal act is present.

Proof of whether the accused was actually in an amnesic state is also sought. Amnesia is not a defense against the accusation of a criminal act, but it may show diminished capacity and result in a less severe sentence. Various states handle the diminished capacity defense differently.

Wolf has recently reported on five young, alcoholic Alaskan natives, each of whom committed a homicide during one of his many blackouts. During experimentally induced alcohol intoxications while in jail, the subjects were unable to recall the homicide or other incidents temporally related to the crime.

They blacked out during the alcohol intoxication test, and the author noticed an abrupt mood change that seemed to coincide with the amnesic episode. The mood shifted from enjoyment to anger, at times associated with overtly violent behavior. The prisoners later remembered their alcoholic exposure as pleasurable because of the lack of recall of the dysphoric mood interval.

Suicide attempts have been reported in connection with blackouts. These are believed to be related to the depressive mood that may occur, the disinhibited loss of control over behavior, and the retention of the physical capability to execute the suicidal effort.

SUMMARY

The presence of a global amnesia for hours or days during and after the liberal usage of alcoholic beverages is an interesting event. That a person without a major disruption of consciousness is unable to remember what happened must be impressive, but apparently most drinkers learn to tolerate such lapses. Serious adverse consequences are possible during the amnestic episode because mood changes and disinhibited behavior can accompany the loss of the ability to lay down recently acquired information. At times, when a criminal act has been committed and the alleged assailant has no recall for the incident, physicians will be called upon to testify on the nature, cause, and differential diagnosis of a blackout.

Blackouts must have a biochemical substrate that would be worth knowing so that our understanding of the process is improved. Furthermore, their prevention might be possible. Since they are fairly well reproduced in those drinkers who routinely experience them, the more thorough study of the alcohol amnestic state is both possible and justifiable. It may also be worthwhile to follow a group of people vulnerable to blackouts in order to determine whether the amnestic-confabulatory syndrome occurs with greater frequency with them than with other alcoholics.

BIBLIOGRAPHY

- Goodwin, D. W. Alcoholic blackout and how to prevent it. In: I. M. Burnbaum & E. S. Parker, eds. *Alcohol and Human Memory.* Lawrence Erlbaum Assoc. Hillsdale, N.J. 1977.
- Goodwin, D. W., *et al.* Alcoholic blackouts and Korsakoff's syndrome. In: M. Gross, Ed. *Alcohol Intoxication and Withdrawal II.* Plenum, New York, 1975.
- Ryback, R. S. The continuum and specificity of the effects of alcohol on memory. Quart. J. Stud. Alcohol 32:995–1061, 1971.
- Tamarin, J. S., *et al.* Alcohol and memory: Amnesia and short-term memory function during experimentally induced intoxication. Am. J. Psychiatry. 127:95–100, 1971.
- Tarter, R. E. & Schneider, D. V. Blackouts: Relationship with memory capacity and alcoholism history. Arch. Gen. Psychiat. 33: 1942–1946, 1976.
- Tarter, R. E. & Sugarman, A. A. Craving for alcohol. In: M. M. Gross, ed. *Alcohol Intoxication and Withdrawal IIIb,* Plenum, New York, 1977.
- Wolf, A. S. Homicide and blackout in Alaskan natives. J. Stud. Alcohol, 41: 456–462, 1980.

15. The Many Causes of Alcoholism

Why is it that of two rather similar-appearing social drinkers, one will continue his modest consumption indefinitely, while the other will come to use increasing amounts and wind up with his drinking out of control and his health, family situation, or his career seriously impaired?

Since there is rarely a single cause for a person becoming alcoholic, the answer is usually complicated. It seems worthwhile to review the various theories that attempt to explain why nearly 10 percent of the drinking class drink in destructive ways, while 90 percent appear to handle their intake satisfactorily.

Causes of alcoholism are usually sorted into three groups: biological, physiological and sociocultural. This classification will be followed here, recognizing that alcoholism is normally the interplay of all these factors.

BIOLOGICAL

Genetic

There are a number of points at which genetic differences can impinge on the drinking pattern.

• A person might inherit a susceptibility to the acute, intoxicating effects of alcohol, so that small quantities produce loss of control over subsequent intake.

• Ethanol is broken down in a series of metabolic reactions. People, perhaps even races, differ in the rate of enzymatic degradation. A genetically determined, impaired ability to catabolize ingested alcohol would be associated with a poor ability to "hold" one's liquor.

• The brain cells of different people may have an inherited, variable ability to adapt to high or chronic levels of alcohol.

• Certain personality features may be genetically determined. In the case of the potential alcoholic, it may be an inherited difficulty in dealing with anxiety, frustration, and depression.

• An organ vulnerability, genetically determined, may make one person more likely than others to develop certain of the complications of chronic alcohol consumption.

A considerable interest in the inherited aspects of destructive drinking is now occupying the attention of certain investigators, especially in Scandanavia. The issue of the inheritance of alcoholic traits becomes a practical matter when counseling children who have one or more alcoholic parents. The well-known fact that excessive drinking runs in families is obviously no grounds for attributing noxious drinking behavior to one's chromosomes. Environmental factors would also play a significant role in such instances. Studies of families of alcoholics always show higher rates among relatives than in the general population, commonly quoted as about 4 percent for men and a half to 1 percent in women. Sons of alcoholic parents have rates as high as 25 to 50 percent, while the rate for daughters is 3 to 7 percent. The environmental factor could be sorted out if the children of alcoholic parents who were adopted by non-alcoholic foster parents soon after birth were studied. This has been done by Shuckit(1) and Goodwin.(2) They believe that genetic factors do play a role in the transmission of an alcoholism potential to the children. In a Danish twin study 25 percent of non-identical twins and 65 percent of identical twins who had at least one alcoholic parent became alcoholics whether they were reared by alcoholic parents or by non-alcoholic foster parents.

This evidence is far from conclusive for a predetermined dipsomania. At most it would speak for an inherited vulnerability to become an excessive drinker, perhaps on the basis of a diminished capacity to tolerate stress. It is therefore not inevitable that a son will follow his father's drinking patterns, especially if he is aware of the predisposition.

Biochemical

Defects in carbohydrate metabolism, for example, a sensitivity to insulin, or episodes of spontaneous hypoglycemia are apparently associated with heavy drinking. Instances of adrenal insufficiency under such conditions have also been reported. However, these endocrine abnormalities are more likely to be the results of unphysiologic drinking practices than their cause.

Alcoholics Anonymous considers the alcoholic to be a sick person whose chemistry is different from others in that alcohol affects him idiosyncratically.

It is true that people vary in their metabolism of alcohol with identical twins having very similar metabolic curves. One study has found that the metabolic pathway in certain drinkers tends to be pushed into anaerobic metabolism. When the anaerobic metabolites combine with acetaldehyde, a product of alcohol breakdown, a compound with a morphine-like structure is formed. This work is far from confirmed, but it has been used to attempt to explain the addictive quality of alcohol.

Endocrine

It is a rather common clinical observation that alcoholic cirrhosis is found in an unusual number of men with scanty body hair. Upon questioning, these people will say that the hair on their chest and extremities has always been sparse. Perhaps, consistently low levels of androgenic hormones predispose to cirrhosis. This finding may indicate that an endocrine basis for some of the complications of heavy drinking exists. In turn, cirrhosis of the liver interferes with the metabolic breakdown of sex hormones, particularly estrogens.

PSYCHOLOGICAL

Tension Relief and Anxiety Control

When people are asked why they drink, a common response is: "Because I feel better; I feel relaxed." In those who are tense under ordinary conditions, or those who are tense because of constant situational pressures, such feelings of relaxation are sought very much. One can visualize that the definite relief from frustration and anxiety, which is often noted from modest amounts of alcoholic beverages, could lead to its excessive use in chronically distraught people. Feelings of guilt, shame, poor self-esteem, depression, and loneliness are soluble in ethanol.

It is interesting that studies done by Mendelson have demonstrated that while small amounts decrease, large amounts of alcohol increase tension states.(3) The heavy chronic drinker, while still conscious, is even more nervous and upset than he was while sober. Therefore, having previously treated one's anxiety with liquor successfully, the search for tension relief can lead to increased drinking. Under these conditions one is driven to drink to the point of unconsciousness.

Personality Disorders

The possibility that some predisposed people have an "alcoholic personality" was once invoked to explain their aberrant drinking. There seems to be no one personality structure involved. Instead, a variety of personality configurations may predispose to a career of alcoholism. The immature, dependent person who does not tolerate life stress well is one sort of individual who may find that drink temporarily solves his perpetual problems. Depressed people, schizophrenics and sociopathic persons are overrepresented in alcoholism statistics. It is more what alcohol does for a person who has difficulty coping than any particular character structure which makes alcoholism a career.

Psychodynamic Formulations

The psychoanalytic literature suggests that alcoholics (among others) are oral dependent types. The orality developed because of deprivation during early life. Some analysts have suggested that alcohol is a symbolic substitute for mother's milk. Their oral dependency is assuaged by drinking, and when they become incapacitated their dependency needs come to have a real, physical basis.

Learning Theory

According to learning theory the tension reduction that results from drinking provides a positive reinforcement to continue to imbibe. The rewards of feeling better, the social approval, one's group endorsement of drinking or of getting drunk all tend to perpetuate the intake of alcohol. When someone abstains after a period of drinking, the shakiness, the hangover, or the impending DTs constitute a negative reinforcement and tend to push the person trying to remain sober right back to drinking. Whether or not one subscribes to conditioning theory, it is important in treatment to know what positive rewards the person is obtaining from drink, and to know what factors keep him from remaining abstinent.

Role Modeling

When a significant person in an adolescent's life relies upon alcohol to deal with the vicissitudes of existence, then the adolescent (whose coping patterns are being formed) may adopt similar unhealthy practices by identification. The opposite can also occur: the young person may be so repelled by the parent's drunken behavior that he develops opposite and negative attitudes toward the use of alcohol.

Traditionally, the family setting was the place where drinking habits were formed. Today, this is somewhat less true. Peer groups make a significant contribution to the formation of drinking practices. Adolescent drinking habits often reflect what the "rest of the kids" are doing. Adolescent alcoholism tends to be an activity clustering among friends. If the gang is involved in heavy drinking or in drugs, it is difficult for any one member to abstain. It is also evident that the adult in certain kinds of work (public relations, for example) is exposed to considerable pressure to drink too much. Some people succumb to alcoholism as a sort of occupational disease.

SOCIOCULTURAL

Culture Specific

Certain cultures (French, American, Irish) have traditionally had high levels of alcoholism, and others (Italian, Chinese) apparently have a low prevalence of alcoholism. A number of reasons for the varying frequency have been offered: The meaning of alcohol in the society, early child rearing practices, or acceptance or rejection of intoxication as a social practice. People living within a culture with considerable pressure to drink and with a high rate of destructive drinking are at great risk. For certain groups in that culture (young, urban males, for example) very heavy drinking is almost the cultural norm. In such a society drinking is equated with manliness; it becomes the way to show group identification and solidarity, and it is the institutionalized way to release inhibitions.

Subcultures under Stress

A subgroup that finds itself overwhelmed with severe conflict in a no-win situation or one living in considerable turmoil will find that large numbers of its members resort to drinking themselves into oblivion as the only way out. Subcultures have been obliterated, in part at least, by alcoholic overindulgence of a major segment of its key people.

ALCOHOLISM: A SYNTHESIS

It seems reasonable to think of alcoholism as the end product of a combination of the various factors mentioned. As a result of their studies, the McCords described a chain of events that often lead to destructive drinking.(4) The following model draws upon their work.

A person with a genetic vulnerability (manifested psychologically or biochemically) had an early childhood of exposure to considerable family stress. This led to an inadequate, erratic satisfaction of his dependency needs, and an inability to form a clear self-image, including a definition of his male role. As a result, he developed intensified dependency needs and was conflicted about the means to satisfy them. As an adolescent he became aware of the cultural pressures as expressed both in the mass media and in daily life to "be a man," and not to be dependent. He therefore adopted an "independent facade" of self-reliance and toughness while still searching to satisfy his underlying dependency.

As he grew up, the pressures for him to accept the independent male role continued. Other alternatives for him to satisfy his dependency needs were not at hand. He found in alcohol a transient release from the underlying struggle between what he was and what he ought to be. Furthermore, drinking was not only culturally acceptable, it was equated with manliness and self-sufficiency, the very qualities in which he felt inadequate. His drinking did not solve the problem, rather it aggravated it. Finally, his tenuous self-image collapsed, his dependency traits broke forth, and his drinking went completely out of control.

Such a chain of events seems to have occurred in some of the children the McCords follow. Other sequences applicable to other men and women, and terminating in alcoholism, also exist. Although one specific event might at times seem to precipitate someone into a life of drink, antecedent factors would surely be required for such a dramatic change in life style.

REFERENCES

1. Shuckit, M. A., et al. A study of alcoholism in half siblings. *Amer. J. Psychiat.* 128:1132, 1972.
2. Goodwin, D. W., et al. Alcohol problems in adoptees raised apart from alcoholic biological parents. *Arch. Gen. Psychiat.* 28:238, 1973.
3. Mendelson, J. H., et al. Experimentally induced chronic intoxication and withdrawal in alcoholics. *Quart. J. Stud. Alc. Suppl. No. 2*, 1964.
4. McCord, W. and McCord, J. *Origins of Alcoholism*, Stanford University Press, Stanford, 1960.

16. Alcohol Withdrawal Syndromes

When heavy and consistent drinkers suddenly stop or markedly reduce their intake, an array of symptoms and signs sometimes emerges. Full-blown alcohol withdrawal syndromes rarely occur in those who have been drinking excessively less than five years.

A well-known precipitant of withdrawal symptoms is severe physical stress such as pneumonitis or a major surgical intervention. Withdrawal, therefore, could be the result of abrupt alcohol discontinuance or the result of physical stressors.

WITHDRAWAL MECHANISMS

The alcohol abstinence syndromes can be conceptualized as release phenomena from the depressant effects of alcohol. Excitatory activity of the central nervous system dominates over CNS depressant activity. Therefore, symptoms such as tremulousness, hallucinations, convulsions, insomnia, delirium, hyperreflexia, and autonomic stimulation become evident. Convulsive thresholds, for example, which were elevated due to the depressant effects of alcohol, are lowered during the withdrawal phase. Similarly, psychomotor hyperactivity is released when the depressant effects of ethanol are terminated.

Other findings are consistently associated with specific withdrawal effects. Stimulation of the respiratory centers as a rebound from the depressant effect of alcohol can cause hyperventilation and respiratory alkalosis during the 48 hours after abstaining. As a result of alkalosis, hypomagnesemia occurs due to a shift of magnesium ions from intravascular to intracellular.

Low magnesium intake due to poor nutrition while overdrinking adds to the low plasma magnesium level during withdrawal. Respiratory alkalosis and hypomagnesemia correlate quite well with withdrawal seizures, tremors, and hyperreflexia.

CLASSIFICATION

A completely satisfactory classification of the alcohol withdrawal states is not yet available. Many atypical and incomplete clinical pictures are seen. Some do not readily fit into current nomenclature. The following categorization does not reflect the highly diverse pathways that withdrawal states can take.

Relative (or Early) Withdrawal

A condition called relative (or early) withdrawal has been described recently. It consists of tremulousness and shakiness upon awakening after a night of abstinence from alcohol. Thus, the morning-after sickness in binge or persistent alcohol abusers can be understood as an early, partial withdrawal syndrome. It is also believed by some investigators that certain withdrawal symptoms build up during chronic heavy drinking and become even more manifest during the post-alcoholic state. These include the sleep disturbances (to be described), agitation, muscle aches, tremors, nausea, tinnitus, anxiety, and depression.

Impending Delirium Tremens

This category includes manifestations such as shakiness, sweating, and low-grade fever. Agitation is not uncommon, and a mild degree of mental confusion may exist. However, when a full-blown delirium, hallucinations, or convulsions develop, they constitute a progression to other abstinence syndromes. Impending DTs is the most common of the withdrawal syndromes. It can begin as early as 12 hours or as late as 72 hours after the last drink. For some people this condition will constitute the entire withdrawal experience. A fewer number will go on from there to the more advanced syndromes.

Alcoholic Hallucinosis

Within a day after drinking has stopped an acute onset of auditory hallucinosis can evolve. It may follow the impending DTs, or it may appear without prodromal symptoms. The sensorium is usually clear and orientation remains intact. The sounds that are heard may be musical, or they may be voices. Frequently the voices make derogatory, accusatory, or persecutory remarks about the listener. The observation that the hallucinated material is auditory and the content is paranoid has prompted some psychiatrists to assume that the hallucinosis is evidence of an underlying schizophrenic process.

Alcoholic Convulsions

Grand mal convulsions without auras can occur 12 to 24 hours after the abrupt cessation of drinking. Both epileptics and non-epileptics may convulse, and a workup for epilepsy is indicated in a person who has his first seizure during withdrawal. Once the person has convulsed, his subsequent withdrawal episodes are likely to be accompanied by convulsions. A third of those who have seizures will go on to develop the full-blown delirium tremens. Status epilepticus is another possible complication in the patient who starts convulsing.

Delirium Tremens

This is a late manifestation of alcohol withdrawal. It peaks three to four days after cessation of drinking. The delirium is a fluctuating type, worse during periods of reduced sensory input. Visual hallucinations are of the homey or occupational type. A truck driver, for example, may vividly describe long journeys along the highway while lying in his hospital bed.

The hallucinations can be distinguished from the abstruse, paralogical hallucinatory activity of the schizophrenic. Stereotyped ideas of alcoholic hallucinations, such as seeing pink elephants, have had little clinical confirmation. The misperceptions are generally frightening, but pleasant ones also have been described. For instance, a drunk tank occupant was entertained over a long holiday weekend by the visions on his private television screen. Marked confusion and variable disorientation are accompaniments to the DTs. The tremors are gross and irregular and become worse when the patient is asked to perform an act. High fever, tachycardia, and elevated blood pressure are associated signs.

The DTs can be life endangering to elderly or seriously ill individuals. With improved treatments hospitals are reporting a less than 1 percent mortality except where large numbers of very ill delirium tremens patients are being treated. Hyperthermia or peripheral vascular collapse are the usual causes of death.

Wernicke-Korsakoff Syndrome

Although not strictly a withdrawal phenomenon, the Wernicke-Korsakoff complex often appears after one of the before-mentioned postalcoholic states. The syndrome is marked by impaired eye muscle control, lid paralysis, deficient recent memory often resulting in confabulation, delusional thinking processes, peripheral neuritis, and ataxia. The condition is sometimes reversible with thiamin and other B complex vitamins. It seems to represent a severe B avitaminosis and, in fact, beri-beri and pellagra may coexist.

SLEEP DISTURBANCES DURING WITHDRAWAL

Considerable research has been done in recent years concerning changes in sleep patterns during heavy drinking and withdrawal. During a binge, REM (dreaming) sleep may diminish, and some intoxicated people might have 0 percent REM time during sleep. During withdrawal, REM sleep rebounds and may occupy as much as 100 percent of sleep time. Some workers believe that the high REM levels relate to the awake hallucinatory activity with postalcoholic hallucinations being a sort of waking dream. Exactly the opposite effect is seen on delta and theta waves (slow waves, or Stages III and IV) sleep. It is increased during the intoxication period and decreased during withdrawal.

Total sleep time may be increased during the intoxication period although sleep fragmentation is regularly reported. Insomnia is a common concommitant of withdrawal. Sleep onset is delayed and multiple awakenings occur. Some patients are afraid to close their eyes because of the horrors (frightening hallucinations). Nightmares waken them from sleep.

A number of clinicians speak of a terminal sleep in which a patient gets a night of deep, refreshing sleep during his DTs. He then awakens essentially recovered from this postalcoholic withdrawal state.

TREATMENT OF WITHDRAWAL

General

Correction of pre-existing malnutrition, avitaminosis, and anemia should begin as soon as oral feeding is possible. A fluid and electrolyte imbalance may exist, but intravenous rehydration must be accomplished cautiously, and the oral route used when possible. Hypokalemia and hypomagnesemia are the most frequent electrolyte abnormalities. Potassium and magnesium sulfate are worth supplying when these deficits exist. A search for infections and injuries should be routinely made.

These patients have a reduced pain sensitivity and poor thermal regulatory capability. Therefore, a serious infection or surgical emergency may be smoldering without being clinically apparent. Those diseases associated with chronic alcoholism must be looked for; otherwise disasters can occur. For example, the patient may seem to recover from his withdrawal syndrome only to become increasingly confused and drowsy. This might be considered a relapse by his physician. There is a possibility that a decompensated liver, unable to handle the protein provided during refeeding, has resulted in aminoacidemia and impending hepatic coma. Other general supportive measures include regulation of urinary and bowel function, correction of hyperacidity, skin care, and oral hygiene.

Preventive

Some physicians routinely prescribe broad spectrum antibiotics when temperatures exceed 101 degrees. Others wait for more definite proof of infection. For very high fevers cooling measures become mandatory.

It is common practice to use Dilantin and phenobarbital or Valium as a prophylactic during detoxification from alcohol. Ordinary amounts of Dilantin orally may not act quickly enough to prevent convulsions. Oral Dilantin in 300 mg doses or intramuscular Dilantin in full doses are preferable.

Large quantities of thiamin and the remainder of the B complex are routinely given to correct a massive deficiency that most alcoholics have and to prevent such conditions as Wernicke-Korsakoff's syndrome.

Soon after mental functioning recovers, the patient should be engaged in conversations leading to a long-term treatment program for the drinking problem.

Sedation

Librium is the preferred drug but other agents such as paraldehyde, the phenothiazines like Mellaril, and the antihistamines like Vistaril also are widely used. The principle is to quiet the patient so that he does not exhaust. There are hazards with these sedatives but the benefits outweigh them.

Sleep is important and chloral or Dalmane are indicated for withdrawal insomnia. They do not produce the same REM disturbances alcohol does.

After recovery, sedatives should gradually be reduced and eliminated if possible. For long-term use, noneuphoria producing sedatives may be preferable in patients prone to abuse substances. Placebos are satisfactory support for a few recovered patients.

Outpatient Management

Hospitalization is necessary for the severe alcohol withdrawal syndromes—particularly convulsions and delirium tremens. If impending DTs exist and the symptoms are mild, and if no significant medical or surgical complications are present, outpatient management can be considered. It is important to see the patient daily and to provide only a day's supply of sedatives. A reliable caretaker in the home is also a necessity.

SUMMARY

The various alcohol withdrawal syndromes described appear as multiple, variegated symptom complexes. If the concept of an early withdrawal syndrome is accepted, then they are frequent. Alcohol withdrawal syndromes are serious medical-psychiatric problems, especially when intercurrent illness coexists. With existing medical capabilities, survival is to be expected in most instances.

BIBLIOGRAPHY

- Gross, M. M., *et al.* Acute alcohol withdrawal syndrome. In *The Biology of Alcoholism,* Eds.: B. Kissin and H. Begleiter, Vol. III, pp. 191–263, Plenum, New York, 1973.

- Gross, M. M., *et al.* Sleep disturbances in alcoholic intoxication and withdrawal. In: *Recent Advances in Studies of Alcoholism*, pp. 317–397, Pub. No. (HSM) 71–9045, Washington, D.C., 1971.
- Mello, N. K. and Mendelson, J. H. Alcoholism: A Biobehavioral Disorder. In: *American Handbook of Psychiatry*. M. F. Reiser, Ed., Vol. IV, 1974.
- Wolfe, S. and Victor, M. The physiological basis of the alcohol withdrawal syndrome. In: *Recent Advances in Studies of Alcoholism.* Pub. No. (HSM) 71-9045, 1971, Washington, D.C.

17. The Management of Acute Alcoholic States

DIAGNOSIS

An obviously intoxicated patient brought in for emergency care often has associated conditions that require diagnosis. Due to his incoordination or belligerence he may have sustained skull or skeletal fractures, a subdural hematoma, aspiration pneumonia, or other injuries. At times a person with alcohol on his breath may be comatose from diabetic acidosis, hypoglycemia, or sudden blood loss from a perforated peptic ulcer or bleeding esophageal varices.

Mixed intoxications are becoming common these days. One author reports that over 25 percent of lethally intoxicated patients had ingested both alcohol and barbiturates.(1) Blood alcohol and barbiturate levels can be helpful in establishing a complete diagnosis. During recovery from acute intoxication or from one of the withdrawal states other serious conditions may become evident. Schizophrenics may drink excessively in a futile effort to treat their emotional disorder. Alcoholic dementia, polyneuritis, or liver insufficiency might become manifest as the acute symptoms subside.

HOSPITAL CARE

A stuporous or comatose patient requires observation and treatment in a general or psychiatric hospital. As a rule a patient does not reestablish physiological equilibrium for approximately 10 days. Occasionally, he may be safely transferred to a Recovery House or Limited Care Facility after a few days. The impending withdrawal state (tremulousness, insomnia, agitation, sweating, rapid pulse) must be evaluated for the need to hospitalize. If hallucinations in any sensory system along with fever, delusions, disorientation, or seizures appear, hospitalization is clearly indicated.

NURSING CARE

Close observation is essential until it is established that other acute medical, orthopedic, or neurosurgical conditions are not present. Heart rate, blood pressure, respiration, fluid intake and output, and level of consciousness should be monitored at 15 to 45 minute intervals until the patient regains consciousness.

Bed rails and other protective devices are prudent. However, bed rails may only increase the height of a fall that a hyperactive patient sustains. A sitter (preferably a close family member) should be available in questionable situations. The sitter will also serve to help the patient interpret reality, and constitute a familiar object in a strange environment.

The room ought to be well-lighted, without shadows or other items capable of misinterpretation. Illusions are more common in a delirium than hallucinations. Anything that can be done to eliminate ambiguous sensory stimuli should be done. For the same reason, communications should be simple and direct.

If the patient is panicky, combative, or hyperactive, chemical restraints are preferable to physical restraints. The latter may be interpreted in a paranoid manner as very threatening. In addition, certain chemical quieting agents have other actions that are beneficial (anti-emetic, muscle relaxant, anticonvulsant, sedative).

MEDICATION

Alcohol is still used, although infrequently, in gradual detoxification. While some rationale for its use exists, other equally effective medications will control the withdrawal symptoms and do not prolong the tissue changes produced by alcohol. Furthermore, by completely eliminating alcohol the impression is not transmitted that alcohol is a treatment for the problem. It is possible to completely and abruptly discontinue the patient's use of alcohol, providing other sedatives or tranquilizers are given when he becomes excited or agitated. Naturally, depressants are not indicated for the stuporous or comatose patient. The parenteral route is preferred when cooperation is impaired, or nausea or vomiting exist.

The drug of choice currently is chlordiazepoxide (Librium).(2) It produces adequate sedation with little risk of dependency. It has some anticonvulsant action and few side effects. This medication can be given in 50-100 mg doses every three to four hours as necessary. In extremely over-agitated patients the

100 mg i.m. dose may have to be repeated hourly once or twice. Care should be taken not to oversedate the patient. Under ordinary conditions chlordiazepoxide can be gradually reduced over three to five days and eventually restricted to a bedtime dose.

If chlordiazepoxide is ineffective or produces some undesirable effect, chlorpromazine (Thorazine) 50-100 mg orally or intramuscularly, or thioridazine (Mellaril) 50-100 mg orally can be given every three to four hours. Paraldehyde is quite effective in 10-20 cc doses orally, but the odor is unpleasant and may irritate the gastric mucosa. It should not be used along with disulfiram (Antabuse).

Hypnotics may not be necessary and should not be used routinely. Chloral hydrate 500 mg or flurazepam (Dalmane) 30 mg can be ordered for sleep and discontinued as soon as possible.

Recent studies indicate that acute alcoholic withdrawal states are often accompanied by overhydration, and it is best to avoid parenteral fluids.(3) Exceptions occur when vomiting, high fever, or diarrhea exist, or when dehydration is demonstrated. As soon as he can swallow, the patient can have fluids *ad lib*.

Certain symptoms of the acute withdrawal syndrome require symptomatic treatment. Severe muscle tremors can be treated with diazepam (Valium) 10 mg every three to four hours. If convulsions occur, diazepam is also helpful. Diphenylhydantoin (Dilantin) has not been definitely shown to be of value. Its onset of action is too slow to be effective in withdrawal convulsions due to alcohol. Some clinicians will administer phenobarbital prophylactically. If status epilepticus intervenes, diazepam is very useful.

Barbiturates can be used for acute alcohol withdrawal, but they should probably be avoided. They produce physical and psychological dependency, are popular agents for suicide, and are no longer necessary now that safer, less addicting drugs are available. If used, they should be discontinued within a week.

It has been fairly well established that hypomagnesemia occurs during the acute states. Whether magnesium ameliorates the symptoms, particularly the tremors and muscle irritability, is not yet proven. The recommended dose is 2 cc of a 50 percent magnesium sulfate solution given intramuscularly every four to six hours. The other electrolytes do not show consistent changes and tend to reach equilibrium as soon as oral intake is resumed.

Vitamins, particularly the B complex, are worth prescribing during the acute and convalescent phases. Parenteral vitamins are not ordinarily necessary.

It is well for the physician to learn a standard detoxification procedure for routine use and modify it for special situations. With present-day management of the acute alcoholic states, the mortality rate has decreased. When delirium tremens develops, there may be a mortality of about 1 percent or less when proper care is given.

AFTERCARE

It is discouraging how often a patient who has been informed of the consequences will continue to drink after a portocaval shunt or an incapacitating polyneuritis. On the other hand, somatic disease secondary to alcohol might provide leverage for some patients finally to seek help with their drinking problem. By the time their drinking has resulted in organ damage, it is almost futile to expect that they can "cut down" and become social drinkers. The goal should be abstinence for such individuals. Whatever persuasive powers the physician has should be used to induce his patient to enter into treatment with a caregiver now.

While the patient remains in the acute treatment or convalescent hospital, a study of his past drinking patterns and the needs they served should be made. As soon as the patient can cooperate, the damage done to his health, his family, his social and economic status is evaluated, and the picture discussed honestly and without judgmental attitudes. Every patient is entitled to know the consequences of continuing to drink. Some will make a rational decision to seek help. Others will require further proof of their destructive behavior. If an ongoing alcoholism program exists in the hospital, the process of instituting treatment is much easier. The ward routines automatically compel him to attend the educational films, lectures, AA meetings, group therapy sessions, and other elements of the program.

Individual contacts by the professional and paraprofessional staff need not be neglected. Every problem drinker has one or more sensitive areas through which he can be "reached," if these can be found. It may be a highly prized intelligence, the integrity of his body, a beloved child, or a wife on whom he is extremely dependent. Discussions may impel him to make the great sacrifice of relinquishing alcohol if the promise of a greater reward is made clearly visible. The search for such critical elements is an important part of the persuasion process.

The alcoholic during and immediately following the period of detoxification is more amenable to change than on any other occasion. His first episode of DTs or his first hospitalization may be a sort of "hitting bottom." An intense and coordinated effort should be made prior to discharge to ensure the patient's continuation in a therapeutic program. This can be aided by talks with the patient and spouse, a psychiatric consultation, or an introduction to an Alcoholics Anonymous meeting. It is best to arrange for the patient's appointments before he leaves and rely on spouse or friend to help him keep them.

Contact with the patient and support from his physician is helpful until the program "takes." In this way the physician can transfer his rapport and his relationship to the clinic, psychiatrist, AA, or other group program. The physician can then feel he has fulfilled his obligation to the patient and given him an adequate start on a recovery program.

SUMMARY

The management of pathologic intoxication, the delirium tremens, alcoholic hallucinosis, and other acute alcoholic states consists of maintenance of vital functions, prevention of injury, alertness to underlying illnesses, and a restoration of proper sleep and nutritional patterns. Gradual withdrawal is recommended to prevent recurrent, major convulsions and shock. Routine administration of parenteral fluids is not indicated. Immediately following recovery from the acute state may be a propitious time to begin the alcoholic's rehabilitation.

REFERENCES

1. Gupta, R. C. and Kofoed, J., Toxicological Status for Barbiturates, Other Sedatives and Tranquilizers in Ontario: A 10 Year Survey, Canad. Med. Assoc. J. 94:863–865, 1966.
2. Kaim, S. C., Klett, C. J. and Rothfeld, B., Treatment of the Acute Alcohol Withdrawal State: Comparison of Four Drugs, Amer. J. Psychiat., 125:1640–1646, 1969.
3. Knott, D. H. and Beard, J. D., Diagnosis and Therapy of Acute Withdrawal from Alcohol. In Current Psychiatric Therapies; (Ed. J. H. Masserman), Grune and Stratton, 1970.

18. Alcoholics: Can They Become Social Drinkers?

The question is an old one. Chronic alcoholics have spent lifetimes sporadically attempting to moderate their drinking. Dozens of articles have been written pro and con. Few subjects arouse stronger feelings among alcohologists.

On the abstinence side are most clinicians, Alcoholics Anonymous, the National Institute on Alcohol Abuse and Alcoholism (NIAAA), and the rest of the alcohol establishment. Those who make up the pro social drinking group are a much smaller band of treatment personnel and researchers.

THE ISSUES

Most chronic alcoholics show an intermittent drinking pattern. Some are binge drinkers who may only have one or two devastating drinking sprees a year. In between they are dry or drinking moderately.

Even the heavy daily drinker who would go into one of the withdrawal syndromes if he stops will modulate his intake for months after a bout of the DTs, the threat of job loss, or entry into a treatment situation. Such reductions in consumption represent neither recovery nor remission. They are cyclic undulations in the normal course of a chronic, life-threatening behavior. To identify these fluctuations during treatment and call them improvement is a bit naive.

One characteristic of the alcohol dependent person is a general inability consistently to drink moderately. Some are so lacking in control that one drink may mean drinking until unconscious. For others, the dyscontrol is incomplete. They drink without impairing themselves or others for shorter or longer periods of time. Then, at some point, due to some noxious mood, perhaps, their control is lost. These drinkers should seek abstinence as their goal. They have too much to lose and too little to gain from attempts at controlled drinking.

Other common characteristics of many chronic alcoholics are their enormous ability to deny the seriousness of their alcoholism, and a well-developed capacity to rationalize and minimize the consequences of their drinking behaviors. These factors not only bring them into treatment late, but justify their early withdrawal by dropping out and pronouncing themselves cured. These psychological mechanisms also allow them to employ pronouncements in the media about alcoholics becoming social drinkers as a justification to commence drinking again. However, they do not lack for other excuses equally effective.

Are there ex-chronic alcoholics who can learn to drink in moderation? Probably, but they represent a small fraction of the population at risk and they cannot be predictably identified at present. Thus, at this time with our present knowledge, abstinence is the safest goal. In addition, a person who has experienced years of excessive drinking may have a liver that is functioning marginally. For this person the amount of alcohol consumed while drinking socially is too much.

On the other hand, in a culture like ours drinking is a pervasive social custom equated with friendliness, relaxation, and good cheer. Abstinence is not easy under such conditions. Pressures to imbibe are numerous. Most abstainers have made their adjustments to "friendly" exhortations to drink up. For a few, abstinence represents an irritating social exclusion that is onerous. It is these people, maladapted to abstinence, who might benefit if they could drink moderately while retaining control. Therefore research into this issue is justified and may be productive.

THE RAND REPORT

The controversy about post-alcoholic moderate drinking resurfaced recently when a Rand report by Armor *et al.* entitled *Alcoholism and Treatment* was presented to the news media. Among the conclusions drawn was the highly controversial statement that the treated alcoholics who went back to controlled drinking did as well as those who remained abstinent. The reaction was immediate and was generally very critical. Since then, a number of comments both pro and con have appeared in a number of lay and scientific publications.

The report itself deals with data collected previously from eight Alcoholism Treatment Centers funded by the NIAAA. Clients were re-interviewed at six months after intake and, under special conditions, 18 months after intake. The plan called for 2,320 interviews, but only 1,340, or 58 percent, could be found. Actually, most of the statistics dealt with 597 men from the above group. After dividing the group into various subgroups, it appears that the proposition that alcoholics can return to normal drinking hinges upon the results with a small number of clients.

CRITIQUE OF THE REPORT

The long litany of criticisms of the report would fill a textbook on experimental design and methodology. Many technical points will not be included here. Only the major remarks made by those who have commented publicly are noted below.

General

1. Releasing the report to the press before it had been published in a scientific journal or government publication prevented peer review, which might have strengthened the manuscript or assisted the authors in drawing conclusions that fitted the data.

2. As a result of the media's treatment of the report, a few dry alcoholics have resumed drinking, a practice that could be dangerous for them.

3. To make a newsworthy statement to the press such as ''alcoholics can learn to drink moderately,'' and then hedge it with disclaimers is unrealistic. Of course, the media will pick up the statement and ignore the disclaimers.

4. Some clinicians have made the flat statement that they have never seen an alcoholic who could remain a social drinker for a prolonged period of time. Inevitably, they claim, he slips back into destructive drinking.

Specific

1. An 18-month follow-up provides insufficient time to evaluate the recovery status of an alcoholic. Dr. J. A. Ewing, who has done one of the controlled drinking investigations, said, ''In my study, the results looked promising for the first 12 to 18 months. It was only when we did a long-term follow-up ranging from 27 to 55 months after treatment ended that we detected a universal failure to maintain controlled drinking.''

2. The Rand definition of normal drinking consisted of up to three ounces of ethanol a day (ethanol is 190 proof alcohol; three ounces would make 6 or 7 mixed drinks), and up to five ounces of ethanol on any given day (10 or 12 drinks). This is far above the average amount used by American adults and exceeds the established definition of social drinking (2 mixed drinks or the equivalent a day). Three ounces of ethanol is an intoxicating dose for men of average weight. If consumed in one sitting, it will produce a blood alcohol concentration of 0.1 percent, a legally intoxicating level. Typically, drinkers in the study consumed less than these amounts.

3. Using the three ounces of ethanol or less limit referred to above, then more than a third of the clients studied would have to be considered normal drinkers even before entering treatment.

4. It is well known that alcoholics will underestimate the amount they drink when questioned. Nevertheless, the Rand researchers accepted their estimates without attempting to validate them. As much as a 50 percent error could result from this deficiency alone.

5. The use of interviewers, who also have a stake in making the Alcoholism Treatment Centers look good, is likely to produce client information biased in favor of successful outcome.

6. At the six-month interview, clients were asked about their drinking patterns for the month preceding their interview. At the 18-month interview, they were questioned about their drinking during the previous six months. It cannot be assumed, therefore, that normal drinking occurred over the entire questionnaire period.

7. The number of cases in each subgroup was too small to make sweeping generalizations. The six-month study found that 12 percent were normal drinkers. This percentage would fall to 2 percent if dropouts were included, a customary biostatistical procedure. The 18-month study indicated that 22 percent were normal drinkers, but the more appropriate figure is 13 percent if dropouts are included in the failure category.

8. The study failed to inquire into drug-taking activities. A client drinking moderately but also taking sedatives is not better off and may be worse off than before treatment.

SUMMARY

The advantage of the total abstinence approach is that it is safest for most alcoholics. It provides a sharp and clear danger signal the alcoholic can detect: the taking of a drink no matter what the rationalization. It avoids re-exposure to the substance that is toxic for that individual and that may complete the damage of previously impaired cellular function. It eliminates the futile notion that any of the chemical addictions, whether they be tobacco, alcohol, heroin, or sleeping pills, can be managed over long periods of time by cutting down.

The advantages of the controlled drinking approach are that the person can feel more comfortable in social situations and that people who cannot accept abstinence may be provided an alternative form of treatment. There are alcoholics who cannot or will not make it in AA or other abstinence therapies, and they should have at least one opportunity to try a controlled drinking program, if only as a learning experience.

At our current level of ignorance about treating chronic alcoholics, it seems clear that for most clinicians abstinence is a preferable goal.

ADDENDUM

Since this chapter was completed two important documents bearing on the issue under discussion have appeared. The first is a second Rand report (Polich, J. M., Armor, D. J. and Braiker, H. B. *The Course of Alcoholism: Four Years after Treatment*. Rand Corp., Santa Monica, 1980). The authors now state (in contrast to the first Rand report) "This study does not recommend that any alcoholic should resume drinking." In fact, as the patient group was followed after 4 years, many of those who had been drinking moderately after 6 and 18 months tended to relapse.

The second publication is an article (Pendery, M. L., Malzman, I. M. and West, L. G. Controlled drinking by alcoholics? New findings on a reevaluation of a major affirmative study. Science, *217*:169–174, 9 July, 1982). This paper is a careful follow-up of the 20 physically dependent alcoholics who were originally studied by Sobell and Sobell (see bibliography). The Sobells' article on this group of patients was a landmark report since it was the first positive, controlled study comparing the outcome of social drinking vs. abstinence. It had a strong impact on those involved in the treatment of gamma alcoholism (alcohol addiction). It led to a number of alcohol treatment programs that provided training in social drinking by behavioral conditioning techniques.

The Pendery et al. paper restudied the experimental subjects 10 years after discharge from the hospital. In contrast to the success claimed by the Sobells, the Pendery group found that only 1 of the 20 was able to maintain a pattern of controlled drinking, 8 continued to drink excessively with serious consequences, 4 died from alcohol-related causes, 6 were unable to drink moderately over time and became abstinent, and 1 was missing and reported to be disabled due to drinking.

These recent developments reinforce the conclusion that alcohol dependent persons should be counseled to remain abstinent.

BIBLIOGRAPHY

- Armor, D. J., Polich, J. M. and Stambul, H. B.: *Alcoholism and Treatment*. 1700 Main Street, Rand Corporation, Santa Monica, CA 90406, R-1739-NIAAA, June, 1976.

- Bailey, M. B. and Stewart, J.: *Normal drinking by persons reporting previous problem drinking*. Quart. J. Alcohol, *28*:305, 1967.
- Davies, D. L.: *The problem of normal drinking in recovered alcohol addicts*. Quart. J. Stud. Alcohol, *23*:94, 1962.
- Drewery, J.: *Social drinking as a therapeutic goal in the treatment of alcoholism*. J. Alcoholism, *9*:43, 1974.
- Ewing, J. A. and Rouse, B. A.: *Failure of an experimental treatment program to inculcate controlled drinking in alcoholics*. Brit. J. Addiction, *71*:123, 1976.
- Fox, R.: *Behavioral Research, Therapeutic Approaches: Alcoholism*. Springer, New York, 1967.
- Kindall, R. E.: *Normal drinking by former alcohol addicts*. Quart. J. Stud. Alcohol, *26*:247, 1965.
- NCA/ASMA Position Statement regarding Abstinence. National Council on Alcoholism, New York, September 16, 1974.
- Pattison, E. M., *et al: Abstinence and normal drinking*. Quart. J. Stud. Alcohol, *29*:610, 1968.
- Sobell, M. B. and Sobell, L. C.: *Alternatives to abstinence: Time to acknowledge reality*. Addictions, *21*:2, 1974.

19. Problem Drinking in Adolescents

This chapter was contributed by Dr. Richard V. Phillipson, Special Assistant for Medical and Scientific Affairs, Division of Clinical Research, National Institute on Drug Abuse.

With some regularity, older generations have traditionally inveighed against the wanton, drunken comportment of the younger. Therefore, it is with a certain reticence that I report on what appears to be a significant change in youthful drinking practices during the past 25 years.

The situation of ever-increasing numbers of young people abusing alcohol has become so serious that the Secretary of HHS has recently announced a new program costing $35 million to be spent on Special Target Problems and Populations, the first priority of which is youth. In recognition of the extremely severe problem of alcohol abuse among teenagers, HHS has allocated $12.5 million for education, prevention, treatment, and research related to problem drinking among youth in the current fiscal year. In addition, HHS has funded five comprehensive alcoholism-prevention projects, targeted at 75,000 young people, with the help of the Boy Scouts, Girl Scouts, Catholic Youth organizations, and others. In cooperation with the Department of Transportation, the national media, and the alcohol beverage industry, HHS has launched an "information campaign" focusing on auto safety and encouraging sensible attitudes toward drinking among young people.

Today, alcohol-related accidents account for more than 10,000 deaths each year in the age group 15 to 24 years and are the leading cause of death for this age bracket in the United States. In addition, more than 40,000 young people are injured every year in drinking and driving accidents—many of them crippled, paralyzed, or otherwise disabled for life.

WHY IS THIS HAPPENING?

Teenage drinking is part of a larger pattern of increasing consumption of potable spirits that has become worldwide during the past quarter century. In the United Kingdom, for example, the annual per capita consumption rose between 1949 and 1974 by 47 percent for beer, over 200 percent for distilled spirits, and 284 percent for wine. There is a strong correlation between per capita use and alcohol-related problems. For cirrhosis the correlation is as high as 0.98 in Great Britain. For 20 other countries the per capita cirrhosis correlation is 0.94. In those rare instances when the per capita consumption dropped (as during Prohibition in the United States or during the two World Wars in France), the incidence of cirrhosis also fell.

The past quarter century has generally been a period of steady economic expansion and improved living standards, although not necessarily a time of tranquility. In terms of the time worked for each unit of such beverages, the cost of beverage alcohol has been reduced by at least 50 percent, while for most foods the cost has increased considerably. A gallon of milk and a gallon of wine now can be purchased for the same price. It has also been an era of relaxation of controls over the sale of alcoholic beverages for young people.

Easy availability is, of course, only a fragment of the story. Most youth has been increasingly deculturated from family influences and more responsive to peer values and behavior. Youthful disenchantment with established moral attitudes has been the hallmark of the recent past. The upsurge in drug taking of all sorts has not diminished; on the contrary, it has increased adolescent alcohol consumption. Boredom and the lack of meaningful activities contribute to the abuse of alcohol.

More excessive alcohol use by the adolescent can be understood as an adaptive effort. It is an attempt to insure friendship bonds, cope with tension and the conflicts of growing up, deal with unpleasant situations at home, in the school, or elsewhere, and solve the array of problems that confront the young person. It is a tactic of adapting to inner tumult and external difficulties. That it does not solve the problem—that it is simply evasive—does not reduce the attractiveness of the intoxicated state.

Furthermore, we have made no significant advances in the prevention or treatment of young problem drinkers, nor are any breakthroughs perceptible in the near future.

IS THERE AN ADOLESCENT DRINKING PATTERN?

Young people tend to drink less consistently than older people, but when they do drink they consume larger amounts. Therefore, they will be involved with the consequences of acute intoxication (violence, accidents, coma, etc.) more frequently than with the long-term effects of alcoholism.

HOW CAN A PARENT TELL WHETHER A SON OR DAUGHTER IS GETTING INTO TROUBLE WITH ALCOHOL?

Warning signs are not different than those noted in adults: frequent intoxications, accident-proneness, impaired school or work performance, hangover, poor appetite, police problems, and a deterioration of personal and social habits.

WHAT ABOUT ALCOHOL-DRUG COMBINATIONS?

Multiple-drug abuse in teenagers with alcohol as the basic or as a subsidiary drug is a common form of substance abuse. The combination of wine or beer with sleeping pills or tranquilizers is particularly hazardous because of the super-additive effects.

SHOULD CHILDREN BE TAUGHT SOCIAL DRINKING AT HOME?

There has been a fair amount of pressure recently to make it respectable to give drink to one's young children in order that, from an early age, they may grow up to seek drinking as part of family or group activity, to be taken for granted rather than be something special, and, in general, to demystify the whole drinking experience. In an ideal world this would be fine. Unfortunately, many parents are far too confused and guilty about their own drinking to transmit anything beyond their own ambivalence. For those parents whose own attitudes toward alcohol are reasonable, the transmittal of these values can be helpful. In homes where the parents or children prefer abstinence, such instruction, of course, is unnecessary and undesirable.

SHOULD SCHOOLS PROVIDE EDUCATIONAL INFORMATION ABOUT ALCOHOL AND ITS USE?

In order to help demythologize drinking, information about alcohol can be given within the context of a general health course. The difference between social drinking and destructive drinking should be pointed out. The fact that drinking does not make a young person manly or womanly can be emphasized. Hopefully, unhealthy, irresponsible drinking practices will be avoided through exposure to factual material about our national intoxicant. It will take more than the efforts of the schools to finally demolish the fiction that excessive drinking is a pattern of prestige or that it is a necessary part of socializing. It will require a revision of the media's outworn stereotypes. Television, in particular, has much to do in this regard.

WHAT IS KNOWN ABOUT SEXUAL ACTING OUT AND VIOLENCE IN CONNECTION WITH TEENAGE INTOXICATION?

Some youngsters use alcohol to dissolve their superego, to reduce their social inhibitions and gather the "courage" to attempt sexual activities that would have been difficult to achieve while sober. In a similar manner alcohol intoxication impairs judgment, diminishes controls over behavior, increases impulsivity, and impairs skilled motor functioning. As a result violent and assaultive behavior is frequent, including gang-type aggressiveness.

WHAT CAN BE DONE?

In addition to developing effective early training, education, and prevention techniques, the most manipulative variable in dealing with adolescent alcohol abuse is to decrease availability. Alcoholic beverages are so pervasive in this society that making it more difficult to obtain seems hardly possible. In fact, there is a countertrend: the production of sweet wines and sweetened milk-based beverages with alcohol added. These are attractive to juveniles because of their taste. Nevertheless, making beverage alcohol relatively more difficult to obtain, especially among teenagers, might decrease a measure of the harmful drinking practices.

WHICH TREATMENT METHOD IS PREFERRED FOR THE YOUNG ALCOHOLIC?

Group therapies are among the most frequently used techniques with or without AA. Individual therapy may be needed when a serious emotional disorder underlies the drinking problem. Antabuse has a lesser role to play, but may be helpful until new patterns of living are established.

IS IT TRUE THAT ALCOHOLIC PARENTS TEND TO HAVE ALCOHOLIC OFFSPRING? ARE THE CHILDREN OF ABSTINENT PARENTS ABSTAINERS?

Alcoholic parents can lead their children into unhealthy drinking habits, but they also may serve as an example that no young person will wish to follow. Therefore, some children of alcoholic parents grow up total abstainers. A parental example of complete abstinence might be followed by the children, but can, if too strict, lead to alcohol abuse as a reaction to the overly rigid restrictions on the adolescent. A vulnerability to alcoholism appears to be an inherited trait, and young men and women who have parents with severe drinking problems should be particularly careful about their use of alcohol and alcohol's easy availability.

ARE SPECIAL TREATMENT OPPORTUNITIES AVAILABLE? HOW MANY ADOLESCENT ALCOHOLICS GO ON TO CHRONIC ADULT ALCOHOLISM?

Special AA groups have been formed for young alcoholics, and even a few adolescent alcohol detoxification centers are in existence. Cirrhosis of the liver, which takes at least ten years of heavy drinking to acquire, is increasingly seen in patients in their 20s. Since the habits of a lifetime are often formed during adolescence it is believed that many young people with a drinking problem will go on to excessive adult drinking patterns.

SUMMARY

Because of our relative prosperity and the easy availability of alcohol, adolescent alcohol abuse is a growing phenomenon. The increasing use of drink in connection with every social occasion and the requirement that young people keep up with their peers in their drinking practices inevitably lead to heavy drinking. Since all are drinking equally heavily, no one identifies himself or herself as drinking too much. It is therefore concluded that over many years the psychologic and physiologic complications of alcohol will increase.

BIBLIOGRAPHY

- Alcohol and Health: *The Third Special Report to the U.S. Congress,* U.S. Government Printing Office, Washington, D.C., 1979.
- Davies, J. and Stacey, R. *Teenagers and Alcohol: A Developmental Study in Glasgow,* Vol. II, Her Majesty's Stationary Office, London, 1972.
- Edwards, G. Public health implications of liquor control. Lancet 1:424, 1971.
- Edwards, G. and Grant, M. *Alcoholism: New Knowledge and New Responses.* Croom Helm, London, 1977.
- Kendall, R. E. Alcoholism: A medical or a political problem. British Medical Journal. 1:367–371, 1979.
- Rouse, B. A. and Ewing, J. A. College drinking and other drug use. In: *Drinking-Alcohol in American Society.* Eds. J. A . Ewing and B. A. Rouse, Nelson-Hall, Chicago, 1978.

20. The Treatment of Alcoholism: Does It Work?

An article was published that has troubled certain members of the alcohol treatment establishment. It concluded, with qualifications, that our usual package of treatment of alcoholism gave no better results than a minimal treatment exposure.

Administrators and directors of alcohol programs were concerned that the article might be used as an excuse for cutting treatment funds by legislators. Others, who were sure their brand of treatment was effective, could not accept the results.

The final effect of the report, however, will be salutary for a number of reasons. It will impel us to take a more critical look at the existing treatment procedures. And it will force us to look more closely at the diagnosis of alcoholism and alcohol addiction.

METHOD

The article in question appeared in the May, 1977, issue of the *Journal of Studies on Alcohol.*(1) Griffith Edwards and his associates presented a controlled trial of a one-year course of treatment as compared to a single advice-giving interview. The research involved 100 married, male, working alcoholics who, because of their serious drinking problem, were referred to the outpatient clinic of the Addiction Research Unit, Institute of Psychiatry in London. What Edwards and his colleagues did was to select those patients between 25 and 60 years of age who lived within a reasonable traveling distance of the clinic. In addition, those with serious physical or mental diseases were eliminated.

Two groups of 50 patients were formed. They were matched by occupational level and by the severity of their drinking. Assignment to the two groups was made randomly. When the *treatment* and *advice* groups were examined for the demographic variables, no significant differences could be found between them.

All of the patients and their wives were carefully assessed. The patient's history, physical and laboratory examinations, and psychiatric, psychological, and social work interviews were obtained. In a session with the patient and spouse the psychiatrist indicated that alcoholism was the problem, that total abstinence should be the goal, that work should be continued or resumed, and that they should attempt to keep the marriage viable.

Those in the *advice* group were further told that the responsibility to maintain sobriety was theirs. It was then indicated that the patient would not be offered a further appointment but that someone would visit the wife each month to obtain information about the patient's status. It was stressed that if withdrawal symptoms were to occur, a general practitioner should be contacted for help. No medication was given.

The *treatment* group, on the other hand, was offered an introduction to AA, a prescription for calcium cyanamide (an Antabuse-like drug), and medication to take in case withdrawal effects appeared. A further appointment with the psychiatrist was arranged, during which a treatment plan was developed.

The social worker arranged to see the wife on a monthly basis to deal with current problems and to obtain information on progress. Outpatient care was provided, and if that proved unsuccessful, the patient was offered hospitalization with an expected stay of six weeks. The hospital program involved detoxification, group therapy, occupational therapy, and the ward milieu. Joint sessions with husband and wife were arranged when indicated. If an appointment was missed, another was offered.

Although some *advice* group patients sought help from other sources, and some *treatment* group patients engaged in only a minimal degree of contact with the Addiction Research Unit, the overall between-group differences in exposure to treatment was substantial. For example, the time spent in a psychiatric hospital was significantly greater for the *treatment group* ($p < .01$). The *advice* group patients tended to obtain brief admissions (mean = 5.2 days) to a hospital for emergencies or detoxification. The *treatment* group patients generally were admitted for a longer period (mean = 23.9 days) and engaged in a planned alcohol treatment program.

One year after the original intake interview all couples were seen for a final estimate of the patient's status. The monthly records of the social worker and psychiatrist were evaluated for changes in drinking patterns and for success in dealing with personal and social problems.

RESULTS

When the two groups were compared at the end of a year, no changes of significance were found between them. From the reports by the wives, it was found that 37 percent of the *advice* group and 38 percent of the *treatment* group had few or no drinking problems. The wives' reports also showed that 39 percent of the *advice* group and 50 percent of the *treatment* group had moderately or distinctly improved their drinking patterns. Fifty-seven percent of the patients in the *advice* group and 65 percent of the *treatment* group reported a slight or no drinking problem. Fifty-nine percent of the *advice* group and 63 percent of the *treatment* group reported improvement in their drinking patterns. The analysis of the monthly reports of drinking behavior during the year revealed no difference between the groups. The measures of social adjustment also were not significantly different.

When the patients were asked to which factors they ascribed their improvement, 54 percent of the *advice* group and 27 percent of the *treatment* group stated that changes in external realities (working, housing) were responsible ($p < .01$). All other reasons given were non-significant. A surprisingly large number—41 percent of the *advice* group and 29 percent of the *treatment* group—said the initial clinic intake interview was a factor that assisted in their improvement.

CONCLUSIONS AND RECOMMENDATIONS

The conclusion drawn by Edwards was that minimal treatment interventions gave as good results as a conventional treatment regimen in this special population of married men. The quality of treatment offered was considered to compare favorably with those in other alcohol clinics in England and abroad.

Edwards pointed out that certain other studies have shown similar results. He also cautioned against extrapolating these data to other kinds of patients.

Recommendations derived from the study are: (1) that a comprehensive assessment for treatable medical-psychiatric problems take place at the outset, (2) that first aid and counseling be readily available for the alcoholic, (3) that inpatient care be utilized for withdrawal or other serious illnesses, (4) that new treatment techniques be devised that will provide improved results, (5) that studies be made of helpseeking behavior by patients, and (6) that preventive efforts be intensified.

CRITIQUE

This is a well-designed and executed study. A number of technical objections could be made, and some of the more pertinent will be noted, but it would be preferable to accept the general validity of the conclusions and constructively attempt to benefit from the investigation by deriving further testable concepts and strategies.

Insofar as specific criticisms of the Edwards' research is concerned, a number of points can be mentioned. A double blind study would have been helpful in avoiding observer bias, but it would have been difficult to execute. It is regrettable that the study ended after one year of treatment. A post-treatment followup might have been helpful in extracting differences between the two groups.

Matkom (2, p. 1827) points out that the assumption that the more treatment a patient obtains, the better he should respond is not correct. In an open situation the sicker patients will tend to seek more intensive care and yet will respond less favorably. He also notes that the *treatment* group may have been more seriously ill than the *advice* group. Thirty-two percent of the *treatment* group as contrasted to 22 percent of the *advice* group had reported prior inpatient treatment for alcoholism.

The *treatment* group also had averaged 16.2 weeks off work during the year preceding the study (approximately 31 percent) as compared to 12.4 percent for the *advice* group. While these figures did not achieve statistical significance, the trend favored the *advice* group.

Schuckit (2, p. 1813) states that a third to a half of all alcoholics will be abstinent or almost so at some particular time. Further, a quarter to a third of all alcoholics also can be expected to cease drinking at some time during their lives even without treatment. If these facts are not considered, they may wash out significant differences between treatment vs. non-treatment groups.

The study under consideration gives further support to the idea that alcoholism is not a single disease entity but rather a multiplicity of disorders. If this is so, then a standard treatment, however effective for certain patients, must surely fail when all alcoholics are assigned to it. The analogy with pneumonia is cited by Glaser (2, p. 1819). If penicillin were considered the usual treatment for pneumonia, then those with pneumococcal pneumonia would be helped. But many others—those with staphlococcal pneumonia, for example—would not respond at all. There are many alcoholisms just as there are many pneumonias. The vast personality differences, the variations in drinking intensity, and the dissimilar life situations make a single categorization for therapeutic purposes unjustifiable and counterproductive.

If alcoholism is a heterogeneous condition, then the "average package of help" is inappropriate treatment and will be found to be no better than minimal treatment. The small number who benefit from it will be canceled out by the majority who remain unaffected.

Glaser suggests a "matching hypothesis" for alcoholism. Alcoholism should be considered multiple diseases with multiple causes, drinking patterns, and character structures involved. If this is so, then differential treatment programs designed for each person are required for optimal management. "Does treatment work?" becomes a meaningless question. Instead, "What treatment, by whom, is most effective for this specific individual with his special problems?" becomes the proper question to study.

Assuming this diagnostic plurality to be true, then the prime needs of an effective alcohol treatment program would be (1) meticulous evaluation, (2) skillful triage or sorting, and (3) a broad variety of treatment options. Of course, the notion of "the alcoholisms" is not new, neither is the concept of matching patient to treatment. These concepts are generally acknowledged but their translation into action is not consequentially executed.

Certain other implications that derive from Edwards' provocative article can be mentioned. Perhaps more emphasis should be placed on assigning the responsibility for one's own cure to the patient. The statement about personal responsibility for one's recovery to the *advice* group may have been more therapeutic than was recognized. We also should look into the therapeutic impact of a thorough assessment procedure. The patients' comments that they benefited most from changes in their environmental situation ought to be taken seriously, and increased environmental manipulations be attempted and evaluated. Finally, effective treatments that will emerge in the future should not be incorporated into a multimodality package. Instead, they should be used for the selected minority who will benefit most from them.

SUMMARY

When a report that contradicts our strongly held ideas comes forth, it is preferable to study the new information constructively rather than pick it apart to expose its inadequacies. It becomes an opportunity to rethink or retest our position. Even if the report turns out to have certain defects, it should not be discarded or set aside.

The paper under consideration should be read in its entirety and used as a stimulus to improve our diagnosis of the alcoholisms, refine our sorting skills, and improve our treatment efforts wherever possible.

REFERENCES

1. Edwards, G. et al. Alcoholism: A controlled trial of "treatment" and "advice." *J. Stud. Alcohol. 38:*1004, 1977.
2. Kissen, B. et al. Alcoholism: A controlled trial of "treatment" and "advice." *J. Stud. Alcohol. 38:*1804, 1977.

BIBLIOGRAPHY

• Emrick, C. D. A review of psychologically oriented treatment of alcoholism. II. The relative effectiveness of different treatment approaches, and the effectiveness of treatment vs. no treatment. *J. Stud. Alcohol. 36:*88, 1975.

21. Alcoholism and Women

Established stereotypes about excessive drinking by women are, no doubt, based upon valid observations. The suburban housewife, alone, drinking because of boredom and frustration is one such prototype. The menopausal woman whose busy life as a homemaker has suddenly become empty because the children have all left the nest is another.

Newer patterns also are emerging. The liberated young college girl may find herself too heavily into drinking. The harassed executive trying to keep ahead of her job or acting the role of "one of the boys" with her co-workers might slip into a pattern of overdrinking as time goes on.

It is evident that changes in the direction of an excessive consumption of alcohol among certain groups of women are appearing more frequently these days. For this reason a re-examination of the present relationships between women and alcohol is considered worthwhile.

HOW MANY WOMEN DRINK ALCOHOLIC BEVERAGES IN THE UNITED STATES?

As of 1979, 60 percent of American women drank some quantity of fermented beverages (as compared to 75 percent of men). It is clear that these percentages are higher at present, due, perhaps, to the large numbers of teenage girls who are counted as users of some form of alcohol.

HOW MANY ALCOHOLIC WOMEN ARE THERE?

It is claimed that more than two million women are in trouble because of their destructive drinking in this country. The male:female ratio is about 4 or 5 to 1. Chafetz, on the other hand, has reported that there are three million alcoholic and problem drinking women, and that the male:female ratio is 3 to 1.

WHAT CAN BE SAID ABOUT THE PARENTS OF THE ALCOHOLIC WOMAN?

A quarter to a half of their fathers were alcoholics and were described by the women as warm and gentle. The mothers tended to be described as cold and domineering, but few of the mothers were alcoholics.

CAN WOMEN DRINK AS MUCH AS MEN?

Alcohol diffuses rapidly to all tissues, and its effects parallel body weight fairly closely. Therefore, women—who tend to weigh 25 to 35 percent less than men—will have higher blood alcohol concentrations and will be more affected when consuming equal quantities of alcohol. Intoxification will occur sooner, and, on chronic usage, organ damage will develop earlier in women.

HOW CAN EXCESSIVE DRINKING BE DIAGNOSED IN WOMEN WHO DO NOT GIVE SUCH A HISTORY?

In general, the signs and symptoms are similar to those in men. Sometimes, edema of the face, a fine hand tremor, or redness of the palms are seen earlier in women. Cigarette burns on the fingers or upper chest may be a hint that the patient was intoxicated and fell asleep while smoking. The possibility that the patient is alcoholic should be entertained in working up complaints of amenorrhea.

ARE THERE ANY WOMEN ON SKID ROW?

Yes, about 5 percent of the residents are women, and, even under the congested living circumstances, they tend to drink alone. They have no "bottle buddies" as the men do. Their major social interactions occur when they try to obtain drinks or money from the male residents or others transiently in the area.

IS IT TRUE THAT ALCOHOLIC WOMEN ARE PROMISCUOUS?

Promiscuity occurs in only a small fraction of all chronically alcoholic women. Schuckit says only 5 percent can be described in this manner. The rest complain of a diminished interest in sex, including frigidity and dyspareunia. Promiscuous behavior may take place during the early phase of excessive drinking with the alcohol acting to release behavior from the usual ego controls.

WHAT DIFFERENTIATES FEMALE FROM MALE ALCOHOLICS?

Considerable overlap exists, but certain differences also are apparent. Women who are more emotionally disturbed and more depressed than their male counterparts are likely to be found in surveys of unselected samples of alcohol dependent persons. Often they can relate a specific stress that precipitated their excessive drinking activity. This may have been a serious sexual problem, gynecological difficulties, a middle-age identity crisis, loss of a loved one, divorce, or some similar emotionally traumatic event.

Because of the social prejudices against excessive drinking by women, they tend to drink alone and away from other people. They begin drinking later in life than men, but this is becoming less true. Alcoholic women are divorced by their spouses much more frequently than alcoholic men. Women marry men who have drinking problems more often than men marry alcoholic women.

WHAT NEW PATTERNS OF HEAVY DRINKING ARE EMERGING IN THE MORE LIBERATED WOMAN?

For many women their traditional roles are in rapid transition and the rapidity of change constitutes a stressful condition. Although eagerly seeking equality, for some, a certain ambivalence may remain because of their early indoctrination about a woman's proper place. After achieving a managerial or other important post, the pressures to drink more heavily may increase.

If they have inner doubts about their femininity or doubts about their ability to succeed, such feelings of insecurity may encourage overindulgence. As with men, the physical and psychological pressures of a demanding and difficult job may be a factor. Then, the loss of the previously more dependent state, the loneliness of the new life, even the freedom to be able to make decisions—all these may build up and culminate in drinking as a way to cope with their problems. So it is not only the unsuccessful career woman but also the successful one who may be at risk.

Women are more apt to combine sedatives and tranquilizers with alcoholic beverages. The perils of miscalculating the potentiating effects of such combinations on some occasion are a real possibility.

AA is reporting that 17- and 18-year-old-girls with drinking problems are now attending their meetings. They have been steady drinkers for a half dozen years or more.

Some observers believe that the apparent increase in female alcoholism is not so much due to newly addicted individuals as it is that women are more open about their drinking at the present time. No doubt, greater visibility is a factor, but a real increase in alcohol addiction has been demonstrated. Women are appearing much more frequently at alcohol treatment centers. They are coming to treatment for cirrhosis of the liver in greater numbers than ever. Deaths due to cirrhosis in females are being recorded by Medical Examiners with increasing regularity during the past few years.

WHAT ARE THE EFFECTS OF MATERNAL ALCOHOLISM ON THE CHILDREN?

Statistics indicate that the battered child syndrome is much more likely to occur when one or both parents drink excessively. Physical and emotional child abuse with subsequent emotional disorders in the children are documented. As the primary parent, the mother, in particular, affects her growing offspring's development. It is very difficult for adolescents to cope with their mother's drunken comportment.

WHAT IS THE FETAL ALCOHOL SYNDROME?

Chronically alcoholic, pregnant women have a high perinatal mortality rate (17 percent vs. 2 percent in non-alcoholics). The children they give birth to may be mentally deficient, show poor growth and development, and have a variety of congenital anomalies. These include facial abnormalities with small head size, short palpebral fissures, drooping eyelids, and hypoplasia of the face. Joint anomalies, cleft palate, septal defects, hemangiomas, and a long list of less frequently occurring deficiencies have been diagnosed during infancy. It is suspected that many less severely affected offspring with only mild mental and growth deficiencies escape notice and are never diagnosed.

At the 1976 meeting of the American College of Cardiology, the cardiac defects found in the fetal alcohol syndrome were scrutinized. More than half of the children with the syndrome have heart abnormalities. Tetralogy of Fallot, patent ductus arteriosus, and ventricular or atrial septal defects have been diagnosed. A number of these children have required surgery to repair the congenital cardiac anomalies.

The cause of the syndrome is not malnutrition, rather it seems to be the toxic effect of alcohol or acetaldehyde upon fetal cellular and tissue development. At birth, the cord blood alcohol has been shown to be at least as high as the mother's blood levels, and in rapidly growing and reproducing cells, levels tolerated by the adult organism may damage the embryo.

It might be wondered why such an obvious connection between heavy drinking during pregnancy and gross neonatal changes had not been detected long ago. Actually, the older literature does mention fetal anomalies occurring in pregnant alcoholic women, but the strong correlation has not been made until recently.

WHAT IS THE RELATIONSHIP BETWEEN MENSTRUAL DIFFICULTIES AND DRINKING?

In Belfer's study, 67 percent of women who had menses related their drinking to the premenstrual period. Drinking either began or increased at this time. His alcoholic patients were significantly more depressed and anxious than nonalcoholic women. The endocrine changes during the premenstruum apparently intensify the pre-existing mood disorder.

ARE THERE ANY SPECIAL PROBLEMS IN TREATING ALCOHOL-DEPENDENT WOMEN?

Substantial doubts about self-worth and identity seem to be present in such women. It is worthwhile to pay particular attention to the problem of their self-concept and to support and enhance it. Role definition and clarification may be important in sorting out ambivalent feelings. The established therapies, Alcoholics Anonymous, group therapies, and Antabuse are as effective with women as with men. The fact that such women are more depressed than men may require particular attention.

WHAT COUNSELING SHOULD BE GIVEN ALCOHOLIC WOMEN WHO MAY BECOME PREGNANT?

They should be taught that persistent, high levels of alcohol during pregnancy can give rise to serious developmental problems in 30 to 50 percent of surviving offspring. They should be encouraged to use birth control measures until alcohol intake can be discontinued. If a pregnancy occurs, detoxification and abstinence is recommended during gestation. If this is not possible, termination of the pregnancy might be considered.

DO WOMEN ALTER THEIR DRINKING HABITS DURING PREGNANCY?

One report indicates that some pregnant women may reduce or stop their intake of alcoholic beverages on the basis of an aversion for such beverages. Further study of the nature of the temporary distaste is continuing.

SUMMARY

Female drinking practices are changing. They are becoming more overt, more women are drinking socially, and more are drinking excessively. In these respects, they are adapting a "masculine" type of drinking behavior. A recently rediscovered entity, the fetal alcohol syndrome, indicates that heavy drinking during pregnancy can induce a variety of serious fetal disabilities.

BIBLIOGRAPHY

- Beckman, L. J.: *Women Alcoholics,* J. Studies Alcohol., *36:*797–824, (July) 1975.
- Belfer, M. L., Shader, R. I., and Carroll, M.: *Alcoholism in Women,* Arch. Gen. Psychiat., *25:*540–544, 1971.
- Garrett, G. R.: *Women on Skid Row,* Quart. J. Studies Alcohol, *34:*1228–1243, 1973.
- Hanson, J. W., James, K. L., and Smith, D. W.: Fetal Alcohol Syndrome, JAMA, *235:*1458–1460, (April 5) 1976.
- Schuckit, M., et al.: *Alcoholism: Two types of Alcoholism in Women,* Arch. Gen. Psychiat., *20:*301–306, 1969.
- Secretary of Health and Human Services. *Alcohol and Health. Fourth Special Report to the U.S. Congress,* 1981, U.S. Government Printing Office, Washington, D.C.

22. How Social Drinkers Become Alcoholics

The transition from being an abstainer to suddenly becoming an alcoholic is not the usual course. What is much more frequent is that someone who had been drinking moderately for years will shift the pattern of imbibing to one of problem drinking or alcoholism.

Many students of the phenomenon separate alcoholism from problem drinking. Alcoholism is considered to be a physical addiction to alcohol: the build-up of tolerance over time, and an alcohol withdrawal syndrome varying from shakiness to DTs on sudden reduction or discontinuance of alcohol. A strong desire to continue to drink heavily is an associated effect. Problem drinking consists of difficulties in living directly related to overdrinking. Marital, job, social, or health problems are some of the areas affected. Addiction may or may not coexist. In this chapter, alcoholism refers to both problem drinking and alcohol addiction.

It is most unlikely that an alcoholic person deliberately makes a decision to become one. Instead, he or she slips imperceptibly, without conscious intent, into excessive drinking styles that culminate in alcoholism. This transformation period is important to identify by the individual and by the clinician.

People in a pre-alcoholic phase may be able to correct their drinking behavior more readily if they become aware of their progression toward destructive alcohol usage patterns. This incremental drinking mode probably accounts for the majority of alcoholics, and the question is: Can an early warning system be designed that will alert the drinker when he or she approaches a hazardous consumption level?

The problem is not a simple one. It consists of more than a quantitative change in consumption. Some people can be impaired by daily amounts of alcohol that others seem to consume without apparent difficulties. A fatty liver or alcoholic hepatitis may develop in a person whose intake is ''no more than the others in my group.'' In this country many occupational and social groups imbibe rather heavily and consistently. Some of their members will get into difficulties early. Others may go on indefinitely without encountering alcohol-related adverse effects.

Usually, an escalation of drinking practices occurs during periods of increased stress. A few extra drinks are taken to unwind, to forget, or to sleep. (A drink is equivalent to one and one-half ounces of 80 proof whiskey, five ounces of wine, or 12 ounces of beer. They each contain about three-quarters of an ounce of ethanol.) When the stressful period is past, the newly established drinking routine continues. Under conditions of further stressful episodes, alcohol consumption increases again. Eventually, a point is reached when attempts to cut down or stop fail because of early withdrawal symptoms like the shakes or insomnia; these require alcohol for relief.

The pleasures of drinking can have an entrapping quality. The mild euphoria and social relaxation provided by a few drinks produce feelings of amiable fellowship and good cheer. This is an attractive state, very attractive to some, but some people make the error of assuming that the additional ingestion of potable beverages will serve to increase the fun. The memory of the immediate pleasure is of greater importance than the memory of distant bad effects.

With additional amounts, because of the biphasic action of alcohol, the mild and pleasant stimulation changes to an increasing depression and then to a substantial loss of control over behavior. This up-then-down effect of ethanol on the central nervous system also is well known when alcohol is used as an anti-anxiety agent. Initially, alcohol reduces tension and anxiety. As heavy drinking becomes chronic, anxiety levels are elevated. It may be that this increase in anxiety perpetuates drinking in a vain search for relief. Using alcohol to evade an unpleasant reality to forget one's worries, or to achieve mastery over life's stresses usually turns out to be a poor effort at self-treatment that is compounded by the period of intoxication, the post-intoxication ineffectiveness and debility, and the pre-intoxication drive to escape from the consequences.

The dilemma is that the socially drinking individual has few guidelines to indicate that he may be at risk when his drinking pattern gradually changes. If one stays below two drinks a day, and does not save up the drinks to go on a binge, impairment over the years will not occur (Anstie's Rule). But many people in this culture drink more than that and appear to do well. At what point do we approach our personal danger zone? The answer is not entirely in the amount of ethanol ingested over time, but in how and why one drinks and what the effects are.

We must also remember that even two drinks a day are too much for some people. There are those who are hypersensitive to very small amounts of ethanol, reacting with a flush, hypotension, tachycardia, and chest constriction. Then there are the pathologic drinkers who become violent under the influence of one or two glasses. In addition, a long list of drugs interact adversely when combined with alcohol. These range from antibiotics, antihypertensives, and anticonvulsants to anticoagulants, diuretics, sleeping pills, and many other groups. Of course people with peptic ulcer, pancreatitis, or liver ailments may increase the severity of their disorder by exposing themselves to alcohol. Diabetics and epileptics would be unwise to use alcohol if only because of the risk of smelling like a drunk during a period of unconsciousness, let alone the deleterious effects of alcohol in such conditions.

As a rule the shift to dysfunctional drinking is a gradual one. In large doses alcohol is a protoplasmic poison, but the dangerous level varies for each individual. Furthermore, to tell a person who has been regularly taking four drinks a day, and who has crept up to eight a day, that he is at risk will predictably accomplish little. In fact, anger at being unjustly accused, or a complete denial that a problem exists, are the usual responses. The advice is interpreted as nagging and may, in itself, lead to additional drinking. It would seem more desirable for each person who drinks to examine his own drinking practices regularly and be willing to change them if the suspicion of overdrinking is uncovered.

Self-examination should be a part of the drinking person's routine, and every effort should be made to be as candid with oneself as possible. Examples of questions that could be indicative of a pre-alcoholic or an early alcoholic situation include the following.

DO I GET DRUNK WHEN I INTENDED TO STAY SOBER?

This question speaks to early loss of control over one's drinking. The inability to stop, once drinking has commenced, is an ominous sign. Even an occasional loss of control may be a warning signal. Some confirmed alcoholics are unable to stop drinking after a single drink has been consumed.

WHEN THINGS GET ROUGH DO I NEED A DRINK OR TWO TO QUIET MY NERVES?

Using alcohol as a tranquilizer can be precarious because the dose is difficult to adjust, and no other person is supervising the medication.

DO OTHER PEOPLE SAY I'M DRINKING TOO MUCH?

If the negative effects of drinking are evident to more than one person, or to a single person on a number of occasions, this means that one's behavior is exceeding the social limits. It would be well to listen to such comments, remembering that most people are usually reluctant to talk about the drinking troubles of their friends and relatives.

HAVE I GOTTEN INTO TROUBLE WITH THE LAW, MY FAMILY, OR MY BUSINESS ASSOCIATES IN CONNECTION WITH DRINKING?

Being arrested for drunk driving or drunk and disorderly conduct are not reliable early signs of excessive drinking. Only a minority of these acts are apprehended, so it is unlikely that this was the first such offense. Being confronted with difficulties at home or at work also tends to be the cumulative effect of a long series of objectionable behaviors.

IS IT NOT POSSIBLE FOR ME TO STOP DRINKING FOR A WEEK OR MORE?

Resolving to stop and not being able to carry it off would indicate a definite psychological or physical dependence and reflect a serious future outlook. Being able to stop is encouraging, but it does not eliminate the possibility of binge or other types of destructive drinking. Many alcoholics remain dry for long intervals. It is not being able to stop that is indicative of a dangerous situation.

DO I SOMETIMES NOT REMEMBER WHAT HAPPENED DURING A DRINKING EPISODE?

Blackouts due to alcohol consist of variable periods of amnesia for what happened during the drinking bout. They are to be differentiated from passing out into unconsciousness, which is the end state of intoxication. Blackouts, which are complete and cover periods of hours or more, are definite evidences of alcoholism. Passing out is an unfavorable sign.

HAS A DOCTOR EVER SAID THAT MY DRINKING WAS IMPAIRING MY HEALTH?

Although it is now possible to pick up early evidences of harmful drinking, by the time a medical examination reveals abnormalities attributable to alcohol it is clear that continuing to drink as previously will further damage one's health. Abnormalities of amino acid ratios, plasma lipoproteins, or hepatic enzymes are signals that too much ethanol is being ingested for the liver to cope with.

DO I TAKE A FEW DRINKS BEFORE GOING TO A SOCIAL GATHERING JUST IN CASE THERE WON'T BE MUCH TO DRINK?

Assuring oneself of a sufficient supply of alcohol just in case is evidence of an unhealthy preoccupation with such beverages and speaks for a need to feel "loaded" on social occasions.

AM I IMPATIENT WHILE AWAITING MY DRINK TO BE SERVED?

The urgency to obtain a drink reflects a craving. Gulping drinks is another sign of overinvolvement with alcohol.

HAVE I TRIED TO CUT DOWN BUT FAILED?

As with the inability to stop drinking for periods of time, the inability to cut down is a warning that dependence is present or impending. Cutting down successfully, but eventually slipping back up is another sign of possible future trouble.

DO I HAVE TO HAVE A DRINK IN THE MORNING BECAUSE I FEEL QUEASY OR HAVE THE SHAKES?

The relief obtained from a drink after arising is apparently due to the relief of early, mild withdrawal symptoms. Therefore, a degree of physical dependence is present, and this means future trouble.

CAN I HOLD MY LIQUOR BETTER THAN OTHER PEOPLE?

Being able to hold one's liquor is not necessarily an evidence of manliness or freedom from complications of drinking. It may indicate the development of tolerance due to the persistent consumption of large quantities. Although social disabilities may be avoided by holding one's liquor, physical impairment due to the amount consumed is inevitable.

HAVE MANY MEMBERS OF MY FAMILY BEEN ALCOHOLICS?

There seems to be a genetic component to some instances of alcoholism. People whose parents or siblings had serious problems with alcohol have reason to be extra careful of their drinking habits. Not only may there be an inherited vulnerability, but the early life experience of a child of alcoholic parents may predispose to seeking out consciousness changing drugs or alcohol in later life.

The indicators mentioned above are early or somewhat advanced signs of alcoholism. They should be assessed seriously by the individual concerned or by the health professional who is evaluating him. The recognition that a threat to one's future exists is a first step. The second step is taking realistic action on the basis of the threat. The third step is sustaining the new behavior. These steps are the critical blocks in altering the course of destructive drinking: refusal to accept the information, refusal to do anything about it, and refusal to maintain a corrective course of action once it is initiated.

SUMMARY

We have about 10–12 million alcoholics in this country. The human burden of these people to themselves, their families, and the rest of the population is immense. Primary prevention, the education of those not involved in the disorder, will be the eventual solution, but it is a distant goal. It is in secondary prevention, the redirection of those threatened with alcoholism, that will lead to more immediate results. Meanwhile, tertiary prevention, the rehabilitation of the 10–12 million who can be considered alcoholics, must also be carried out as effectively as possible. Alcoholism is the most important drug problem of all from a public health, or any other, point of view.

23. Alcohol and the American Indian

Some of the material contained in this chapter was derived from papers presented by Joan Weibel-Orlando, Ph.D., Alcohol Research Center, U.C.L.A., and from an unpublished report of a field trip by Logan Slagle, U.C. Berkeley.

Very few American Indian tribes had contact with alcohol in any form, and none had knowledge of distilled spirits, until the early contacts with European settlers. Beer and wine were used in a few areas, but only in connection with religious ceremonies. As the frontier expanded during the eighteenth century, traders soon discovered that providing "firewater" to the Indian lubricated the bartering process. Negotiating trade or treaty agreements with intoxicated Indians was a common exploitive process.

It is believed that Indians adapted their drinking practices from the frontiersman and later the cowboy, who tended to drink rapidly till drunk and then exhibit unrestrained or violent behavior. Although many generations have passed since the frontier vanished, it is possible that these role models still influence current consumption styles.

In addition, the intoxicated state may have meshed with the cultural matrix of certain tribal groups. For example, an important component of the Iroquois' traditional spiritual exercises was the achievement of an ecstatic experience. It has been suggested that some of their drive to drink to intoxication and beyond represented a search to achieve an "out-of-body" state. The Sioux sun dance was also a strenuous effort to disassociate, and the "sacred water" might represent an inferior attempt to fill the void of deculturation and a quest for visionary experience.

Whether it was for reasons such as these or because of the loss of self-respect, homelands, or the ancient spiritual solidarity, the Amerindian population has long had problems with alcohol. In an effort to deal with a deteriorating situation, Indian leaders requested a law forbidding the sale of alcoholic beverages to Indians. In 1832 Congress passed such legislation. This early effort at prohibition did not remedy the situation. Bootlegging and other evasive practices quickly arose. It compelled the buyer to consume the whiskey rapidly and completely. Indians never had the opportunity to learn how to drink moderately or to develop social taboos against drunken comportment. In 1953, this discriminating and ineffective law was repealed, and prohibition became a tribal option. It is interesting to note that 70 percent of the reservations have retained the prohibition on reservation property. Its value is open to question.

EXTENT OF THE PROBLEM

The statistics are grim, and the trend shows no evidence of improvement. Alcoholism among Indians is more than two times and maybe as much as four times the national level and is higher than for any other minority group. Accidental deaths are first among the causes of death for Native Americans, accounting for a fifth of all deaths. The Indian Health Service estimates that 75 percent of injuries to and deaths of Native Americans are alcohol-related.

The first 10 causes of death among Indians show 5 that are directly or indirectly due to alcohol overuse. These account for 35 percent of Indian mortality, shortening the life span significantly and causing enormous morbidity. They are shown in Table 23–1.

Table 23–1
Alcohol-Related Causes of Death among American Indians

Cause of Death	Percent of All Deaths of Native Americans	Percent of Deaths That Are Alcohol-Related
Accidents	21.0	75
Cirrhosis	6.0[a]	90
Alcoholism	3.2[b]	100
Suicide	2.9[c]	80
Homicide	2.0	90

[a]Compared with 1.7 percent nationally.
[b]Four times the national average.
[c]Twice the national average.

In addition, alcoholic pancreatitis, heart disease, malnutrition, and peptic ulceration contribute to the number of fatalities sometimes associated with heavy drinking.

Male Indians drink more and have more problems related to drinking, but the female Indian drinking rate is also at a high level. In fact, it equals the male Anglo rate. The incidence of fetal alcohol syndrome seems to be disproportionately high among newborn Indian infants, but additional studies must be done to confirm this.

ETIOLOGIC ASPECTS

It has long been claimed that Indians metabolize alcohol less effectively than Caucasians; therefore they are more prone to develop the social and physiologic complications of drinking. This means that less alcohol affects them more. A number of studies have been done with variable results. It appears that other factors are more important in explaining the physiological and behavioral toxicity.

Since the American Indian is of Mongolian ancestry, it can be assumed that some will have the Oriental flush syndrome (see Chapter 7, "The Oriental Syndrome"). This condition does occur with some frequency in the Indian population. In one study, 50 percent of Cree Indians flushed after a small test dose. The flush is presumed to be caused by high acetaldehyde levels, perhaps because of deficient aldehyde dehydrogenase activity. Since the flush itself is experienced as unpleasant and, in severe cases, is accompanied with asthma and tachycardia, it should be somewhat of a deterrent to alcohol consumption. Although, in a few instances, this may be true, it certainly is not a group protective metabolic aberration. Needless to say, it does not explain the Indian's problem with ethanol.

Cultural, social, and familial factors are more important than biochemical or metabolic alterations. The contribution of idiosyncratic cultural forms to overdrinking is impressive when considering various tribal alcoholism prevalence rates. The Cherokee alcohol-related death rate is only 6 per 100,000. Among the Cheyenne-Arapahos it is 239 per 100,000.

It must not be assumed that Indian drinking patterns are monolithic or uniform. They vary markedly from tribe to tribe. Sixty percent of Navahos are complete abstainers from alcohol. This compares to about 25 percent in the general population. Some of the Plains Indian groups tend to be most involved with dysfunctional drinking practices.

Urban and rural Indians show different patterns of use. The former group consumes less alcohol and displays drinking styles that tend to conform as much to their social class as their tribal origin. Middle-class Indians in a large city drink more like middle-class Anglos than like poorer Indians. It is probable that the social factors that alienate people—like unemployment, discrimination, and transitional acculturation—play a role in excessive drinking behaviors. Those who have neither roots in their traditional Indian heritage nor a stake in the dominant society are at the greatest risk. Among rural Indian alcoholics, boredom, hopelessness, and the periodic need to release suppressed feeling must contribute to their binge type drinking.

PATTERNS OF DRINKING

What follows is a description of drinking patterns that are more characteristic of Indians than of other groups. It should not be viewed as a stereotype since Indians, like all populations, present a wide variety of drinking customs.

Drinking is often an extended-kin, group-oriented activity. Communal imbibing is considered a sign of friendship and cohesiveness. Group drinking, sometimes in the form of "passing the bottle," is a norm. Collections are taken to purchase the beverage, and non-contributors are also expected to "party." In fact, the strong pressures exerted by the group to drink along contribute to the relapse rate of those who are attempting to remain abstinent. Refusing a drink is tantamount to insulting the offerer. Solitary drinking is infrequent.

Drinking starts early in life and may be preceded by sniffing gasoline or other solvent. There is little interference with an individual's drinking or drunken comportment. The point of consuming is to get drunk, so the beverage is ingested rapidly until it is gone or until the user is stuporous. This sort of blitz drinking leads to quick intoxication. Little attempt is made to conceal one's drunkenness; actually, it may occasionally be exaggerated. "Raising hell"— loud, boisterous acting out, accompanied by manifest aggressive and sexual conduct—is common. Despite the apparent loss of controls, efforts not to "mess up" are discernable. When enforcement officials are present, imbibers will "cool it." That this is not too successful is indicated by the finding that 76 percent of all adult Native Americans' arrests are alcohol related. One member of the group may remain sober so that he can drive the others from bar to bar. Nevertheless, the conviction rate for Native Americans driving while intoxicated was 7 times greater than the proportion of Indian drivers in the total driving population. Such "cruising" is commonly practiced in urban situations— especially on weekends. Indian bars are prime meeting and socializing places. They tend to be animated and loud and the patrons socialize more than in equivalent Anglo bars.

This binge type of fast alcohol ingestion overwhelms the body's mechanisms for dealing with ethanol. Very high blood alcohol levels must be reached quickly, providing little opportunity for the user to adapt to the profound psychophysiological effects. Death from alcohol overdose is known to occur under such circumstances, but a more frequent concern is the complete loss of control over behavior.

PREVENTION AND TREATMENT

An important requirement would be an entirely new attitude towards alcohol by the Indian youth. At present, the policy of placing few family and social sanctions on the young person's drinking, the excessive drinking role models provided by older relatives, and the symbolic rewards from drunkenness all contribute to perpetuate destructive drinking practices. An entire generation of children will have to be educated about the self-destructive and genocidal nature of current alcohol consuming styles and provided with alternative forms of socializing and enjoying. Otherwise, the process continues, and a third of the Indian population succumbs to the multiple lethalities of this single drug.

The bulk of the treatment services offered by the Indian Health Service is oriented toward problem drinking and its antisocial and physiological sequelae. Many of these are conventional: detoxification, counseling, AA or hospital care for trauma or medical disorders. Treatment methods have to be integrated into the distinctive Indian tradition and community support obtained; otherwise, intervention is destined to fail.

Detoxification and urban alcohol recovery centers are no more successful than their Anglo counterparts, even when staffed with Indian ex-alcoholics. When they are located in the skid rows of metropolitan areas, they are perceived not as opportunities to recover, but as a chance to obtain the food, medical care, and services needed to rehabilitate enough to venture out on another bout. Another advantage to the consumer is that the time spent in a recovery home produces a decrease in tolerance so that less alcohol will have a greater mind-altering effect.

The traditional AA group conflicts with the Indian tradition of not discussing personal problems and of not confessing in public. A few AA-oriented Indian lodges have employed the stratagem of having alcoholics regale the group with a lively description of their prowess in defeating the enemy—the bottle—just as their forefathers related the dangers and triumphs of the battle and hunting trips.

Treatment methods indigenous to the culture also exist. Some medicine men attempt to instill pride in the tribal heritage as a basis for change toward sobriety. Some are using the root of the trumpet vine as an Antabuse-like deterrent. It is said to make the effects of alcohol less pleasant.

One of the more interesting approaches to the management of the alcoholic is practiced by the Native American Church. One of the tenets of the Church is sobriety, but when someone slips, the peyote ceremony is used as a treatment. The ritual use of the peyote cactus is believed to have lead to sobriety for some members, although statistics hardly exist. What the peyote ceremony contributes is a depersonalized state of great hypersuggestibility, which, when guided by the Road Man (the one who shows the way), provides an experience of self-transcendence and communication with the Great Spirit. Personal problems are not examined. Instead, the supplicant's destructive life-style is clearly seen, either symbolically or in actual vivid pictures. The Right Way is indicated, and if things go well, the alcoholic reforms his life into a more constructive style.

Intoxication has been suggested by some anthropologists, and by no less a psychologist than William James, as an effort to achieve a higher spiritual consciousness, a state that is highly valued in many Indian cultures. If so, alcohol intoxication is a poor one for this purpose. Peyote provides a much more dramatic, palpable, impressive theobotanical experience. It is unfortunate that the long-term results of peyote exposure cannot be reliably determined.

BIBLIOGRAPHY

- Albough, B. J. & Anderson, P. Peyote in the treatment of alcoholism among American Indians. Am. J. Psychiat. 131:1247–1257, 1974.
- Alcohol and Health. Third Special Report to the Congress, U.S. Govt. Printing Office, Washington, D.C. 1978.
- Alcohol and Health. Fourth Special Report to the Congress, U.S. Govt. Printing Office, Washington, D.C. 1981.
- Burns, M., et al. Drinking practices and problems of urban American Indians in Los Angeles. Planning Analysis and Research Institute, Santa Monica, CA 1974.

24. The One-Vehicle Accident

If you are becoming concerned about the increasing number of homicides, consider that more fatal injuries result from traffic accidents each year than from homicides and suicides combined.

Many young Americans lost their lives during the Vietnam conflict, but many more lost their lives during those same years in domestic traffic accidents. It is incomprehensible why so few people become upset about the 45,000 or so who are killed and the hundreds of thousands who are injured in motor vehicle accidents each year. More than a third of these injuries and a half of the deaths are alcohol related. With wisdom and desire, many of these casualties could be prevented.

THE SINGLE-VEHICLE ACCIDENT (SVA)

The single-vehicle accident is a special type of car accident—one in which alcohol and, to a lesser extent, drugs play a significant role. In various studies, 18 to 51 percent of drivers involved in multivehicle fatalities had a blood alcohol concentration (BAC) of 0.1 percent or higher.

As many as 41 to 72 percent of the drivers in single-car fatalities had BACs in that range. These figures are compiled from 12 studies of multivehicular accidents and 17 studies of one-car accidents.

The statistics from a number of states reveal that the long-term trend in SVA fatalities as compared to all auto accidents is upward. In 1951, 25 percent of all automobile deaths were one-car crashes. By 1961, the percentage had risen to 39.6 percent. In 1977, the majority (56 percent) of fatal car accidents were SVAs.

During the last year for which data are available, 1978, the percentage was

61. Therefore, the SVA has surpassed the multiple-car accident as a fatal casualty-producing agent, and its association with intoxication is unquestioned.

Of course, alcohol is not involved in all SVAs. From Table 24–1 it can be seen that other causes exist. However, in 40 to 60 percent of such mishaps, alcohol intoxication and related effects contribute to the accident. It is evident that most of the SVA causes listed under "Driver Failure" can be attributed to intoxication by some substance.

Table 24–1

Causes of Single-Vehicle Accidents

Driver Failure
Driver intoxication (alcohol or drugs or both)
Sleepiness
Excessive speed
Inept driving skills
Operator distraction
Illness (pain, stupor, syncope, seizure)
Impaired visual or auditory acuity
Suicide attempt

Vehicle Failure
Tire blowout
Brake failure
Accelerator jam

Hazardous Driving Conditions
Dangerous roadway
Adverse weather conditions
Sun or headlight glare
Obstacle on road

SVAs tend to occur late at night or on weekends, coinciding with the periods of heavier drinking and fatigue. Frequently, multiple causes are involved in the crash. A speeding drunk driver dozes at the wheel and cannot react quickly enough to prevent a crash. The results of an SVA may be that the car turns over, leaves the roadway, enters a ditch, or water, goes up an embankment, or hits another object—such as a pedestrian, a cyclist, another vehicle on the road, or a train.

The role of alcohol in SVAs is obvious. In amounts as low as 0.04 percent (one to two drinks) some mild decrement in psychomotor performance is measurable. The impairment increases in a linear fashion until BACs are reached that are incompatible with the ability to drive. It is believed that SVAs are more serious than multicar accidents because higher speeds are recorded in the former type of accident.

SUICIDE

Suicide has special relationships with both SVAs and with alcohol. People intent on suicide have been known to employ their cars to achieve this end. The self-destructive drive may come forth during a drinking bout; or it may have existed prior to it, and the person used alcohol to reduce his fears and to numb himself.

One estimate suggests that 10 to 15 percent of SVAs have a suicidal intent, although this figure has been disputed as too high by others. It has been found that an unusually large number of holders of double indemnity policies die in SVAs.

A recent report from England indicates that suicide is not a frequent cause of single-car, single-occupant deaths. The highest number of such deaths occurred in the 14- to 34-year age group, whereas the suicide distribution increases with age. The age of drivers who died alone in their vehicle was the same as those in SVAs with other passengers.

The authors concluded that undoubtedly a few single-car, single-occupant accidents were intentional deaths but that the numbers were not large enough to affect the reported suicide rate. Therefore, disguised suicides of this sort do not represent a major contribution to the causes of SVAs.

EPIDEMIOLOGY

From the available information, it is possible to separate two distinct but overlapping drinking-driving populations: the SVA drivers and the multivehicle accident drivers.

Those involved in SVAs are younger, often in their teens or twenties. The age group at greatest risk are those between 14 and 24. The youthfulness of these drivers implies an inexperience with driving and drinking. Another rise in the curve is seen among elderly drivers. Adults between the ages of 25 and 55 have the lowest rates. SVA drivers are likely to be single, separated, or widowed males.

The youthful SVA driver is often characterized as having socially deviant traits as manifested by callousness, hedonism, emotional immaturity, irresponsibility, poor judgment, and the ability to rationalize his destructive behavior as warranted, reasonable, and justified. These personality attributes are sometimes associated with youthfulness, and intoxication tends to exacerbate impulsive, risk-taking behavior.

The fact that a surprising number of SVAs happen during fair weather conditions on straight roads within close proximity to the operator's home indicates that driver failure, rather than the adverse non-driver factors are the important causative elements. It has been found that most of the dead SVA drivers had not used seatbelts.

BLOOD ALCOHOL LEVELS

The high percentage of SVA drivers who had BACs over 0.10 percent has been mentioned. In addition, the average BAC for this group is significantly higher than for the multicar accident group. Drivers between the ages of 40 and 60 had the highest BACs, but they accounted for fewer SVAs.

This negative correlation might indicate that age-related factors such as inexperience or recklessness were more important than the degree of intoxication. An equally plausible assumption is that middle-aged drivers may have acquired some measure of tolerance to the effects of alcohol by regular drinking and were less impaired by it.

SPEEDING

More than half of the SVAs occurred at excessive speeds. The median speed recorded was between 50 and 60 miles an hour. In contrast, multivehicular accidents were most frequently recorded at 40 to 50 miles an hour. Despite the higher speeds, most SVAs took place on roads with lower speed limits than the multivehicular accidents did.

SINGLE VS. MULTIPLE OCCUPANCY

The solitary driver is more likely to become involved in an SVA than the accompanied one. This may be due to the restraining effects of the other occupants upon obviously unsafe driving practices. Uncertainty exists in the literature regarding accidents involving one or multiple occupants in an SVA. One report cites a 250 percent greater frequency of unaccompanied over accompanied drivers. In a study of 15- to 19-year-olds in SVAs, only one-quarter of the SVAs occurred when the driver was the sole occupant of the car. Obviously, more information is needed.

SUMMARY

The single-vehicle accident is becoming an increasingly important cause of autocide, injury, and destruction. It now accounts for a majority of motor vehicle deaths. Alcohol is an important factor in these crashes. Youthful drivers are at particular risk. By far, most one-car accidents result from driver failure. Therefore, preventive strategies must include efforts to change the driving behavior of the drinker.

When it becomes generally understood that consumption of even social amounts of alcoholic beverages causes some impairment of driving skills, perhaps fewer drinkers will drive. Consistent and stringent enforcement policies equitably carried out will discourage others who persist in driving after imbibing. Whether raising the drinking and/or the driving age would make a significant impact should be studied.

BIBLIOGRAPHY

- Huffine, C.L. Equivocal single auto fatal traffic accidents. Life Threatening Behavior 1:83–95, 1971.
- Jenkins, J. and Salisbury, P. Single car road deaths—disguised suicides? British Med. J. 281:1041, 1980.
- Krantz, P. Differences between single and multiple automobile fatal accidents. Accid. Anal. & Prev. 1:225–236, 1979.
- Schmidt, C.M. Suicide by vehicular crash. Am. J. Psychiat. 134:175–178, 1977.
- Technical Support Document. Third Special Report to the U.S. Congress on Alcohol and Health. U.S. Government Printing Office, Washington, D.C. 20402, 1978. Stock No. 017-024-00892-3.

III

ALCOHOL/DRUG RELATIONSHIPS

It is no longer clinically desirable to discuss the drug alcohol without including its interactions with other drugs. The abuse of multiple drugs with alcohol is common; alcohol remains a basic substance upon which a variety of other drugs is overlaid. Furthermore, the pharmacology of alcohol is such that it is affected by and affects the actions of many classes of drugs.

The abuse of all mind-altering substances has certain common patterns: intoxication, overdose, withdrawal effects, tissue damage, and so forth. These communalities should be perceived along with the major differences that exist among the various drug classes.

In this section, the similarities, differences, and various interrelationships between alcohol and other drugs are considered.

25. The Now People: Sketches of Lethal Drug Use

An almost exclusively human trait is to look ahead, to include estimates of the future in our present plans and acts. That future may only be as distant as tomorrow for some, while others may think in terms of 20-year plans and beyond.

A related human characteristic, widely shared by other species, is the desire to survive—the so-called survival instinct. Future orientation and survival are so deeply ingrained in our conceptual style that we are hardly aware of them. When we come upon instances of overt self-destructive behavior, they are often difficult to understand and impossible to explain.

On the other hand, it's not possible to lead a completely safe life. A wide variety of not-so-safe activities is indulged in by all. Every day we take a series of low-grade risks; without them life would be intolerably boring or almost impossible. We cross streets, ride in cars, fly in airplanes, climb ladders, and engage in contact sports. It might be assumed that spending one's life in bed may constitute the optimum in playing it safe, but cardiac physiologists tell us that the completely sedentary life also has its dangers.

Then there is a group of high-risk takers who willingly expose themselves to danger for the exhilaration or other rewards of the risk taking. Included in these are the sky divers, the motorcycle and car racers, members of bomb disposal units, and persons who knowingly engage in hazardous avocations or vocations for money or fun.

So we all live in ways that will predictably shorten our life-span. Many of our habits of eating, drinking, smoking, and other ventures are not likely to procure the longest possible survival. Lack of exercise, obesity, overdrinking, and heavy smoking are fairly likely to shorten one's existence, but fair numbers of us seem willing to accept that contingency. This disregard for longevity is probably a result of the delay in the perceived result. Disregarding the possibility of a shortened existence is not hard if the ultimate consequences are years away. Couched in terms of learning theory, consequences that are immediate and pleasurable or pain-relieving are much more reinforcing of behavior than consequences that are distant or aversive.

THE NOW PEOPLE

Over and above the "normal" disregard for maximal survival, certain people seem to have little or no concept of a personal future. They become involved in life-threatening behaviors because they cannot conceive of their own cessation. In general, adolescents tend to be now-oriented, and often behave as though they were immortal. In fact, the end of psychological adolescence may coincide with the first shocking awareness of one's own mortality. A few adults never seem to have acquired this insight and continue to act as though they were imperishable. Their life-style reflects a singular lack of concern about their continuance.

Then there are those who exist without a viable future. In reality or in their fantasy—it doesn't matter which—they are without hope. Their emotional condition ranges from dysphoria to aphoria. Such noxious feeling tones demand relief, no matter that the relief is achieved at a perilous price.

Finally, the now people include those who have been tricked into futurelessness. Some chemical, taken over time, reduces or obliterates the ability to know the consequences of its continued consumption. Alternatively, one may become locked into a drug's repetitious use because of the withdrawal sickness, which is so easily relieved by the substance that caused the sickness. It is fascinating to observe certain otherwise thoughtful people advocate the right to unlimited access to all drugs as a basic freedom when, in fact, dependence on certain drugs drastically impairs or abolishes one's freedom of choice.

It is not surprising that a number of the now people eventually seek out certain mind-altering drugs that will make them feel better than they do. It is also not surprising that such drugs will be excessively used, either because the degree of relief provided is great, or because the usual internal constraints and cultural taboos hardly exist for these people.

The now people do not see any reason why they should not continue to use drugs and why they should not use as much as they need to provide hyperphoria. They are not the experimenters or the recreational users of drugs. They make a career of their substance abuse. They are the rumheads, the potheads, the pillheads, and the hopheads. And their inordinate drug consumption serves to reinforce their futurelessness.

LETHAL PATTERNS OF DRUG ABUSE

Most drug abuse has no lethal intent. Non-medical drug users as a group are quite concerned about their viability and survivability.

A recent example of their concern for themselves was the loud outcry about Mexican marihuana being contaminated by the herbicide paraquat. In fact, there has not yet been a substantiated instance of paraquat toxicity due to marihuana use. That whole uproar was a tempest in a waterpipe, more political than pathological.

But there are certain highly hazardous drug-using practices. Some of them are well known; some are insufficiently documented because the research has not been done, but the street reports are ominous. It is a remarkable commentary on our alleged "instinct for survival" that these precarious patterns of drug abuse are not too uncommon. A number of them are mentioned here to illustrate the self-destructive inclinations of those who have, for one reason or another, little concern about their future.

THE END STAGE, ACTIVELY DRINKING ALCOHOLIC

The person in or verging on liver failure who continues to drink is unquestionably hastening his demise. By this time he must have repeatedly been told of the grim consequences of the continued ingestion of alcoholic beverages. People who have had portocaval shunts for bleeding varices or ascites have been known to continue to imbibe.

I can think of at least one person with a severe alcoholic peripheral neuritis that rendered him incapable of walking, who managed to roll his wheelchair to the nearest liquor store for a daily jug of wine. Then there was the relatively young man with recurrent bouts of acute alcoholic pancreatitis associated with excruciating abdominal pain who would resume drinking shortly after discharge from the hospital. One might have thought that the immediate and obvious threat of dying or of inordinate suffering would be a deterrent. But it was not.

THE PHENCYCLIDINE FREAK

PCP ("Angel Dust") is a rather mediocre euphoriant, but it is widely available, and the price is right. As a result, the young in mind who are despairing, distraught, distressed, desolate, or depressed have come to use the drug often and in increasing amounts. Too often, one of a variety of lethal sequallae emerges. Overdose with death from recurrent seizures or respiratory failure is one possibility. Accidental drowning from loss of orientation, sometimes in small amounts of water, is another. A third is violence to oneself or to others, or deadly force used upon the "dusted" person whose aggressiveness induces counterviolence. A suicidal depression can emerge after partial recovery from a major phencyclidine reaction.

One of the strangest of Angel Dust-related phenomena is the repeated use of the drug after experiencing a devastating, schizophrenic-like psychosis. It is not a rarity to find that after recovery from one or more psychotic episodes of many weeks' duration, the person decides to continue to use the drug despite the previous devastating experience with it.

THE HOT SHOT

When a heroin user overdoses, it is not unusual for junkies who become aware of the event to try to seek out the pusher who sold the material. They assume that the quality of the heroin must be better than the usual street junk, and they want some. The possibility that they might also OD doesn't seem to deter them.

INHALING THE COMMERCIAL SOLVENTS

The abuse of a drug that has been tested for safety and has been used in medicine is one thing. To sniff organic solvents that have never been meant to be used by man or beast reflects a profound disinterest in survival. Not only the solvent, but also the impurities and the active ingredients may be toxic. Such exotic items as insecticide spray, liquid shoeshine polish, transmission fluid, and metallic paint aerosols are in favor in certain parts of the country. Even relatively nontoxic solvents can cause death by asphyxiation when sniffed in an enclosed space or by "sudden sniffing death," when inhalation is combined with physical exertion. Now people are never deterred from using dangerous drugs by giving them information about the possible consequences.

SPEED ROULETTE

As the intravenous speed scene was drawing to a close, about 1970, an occasional tale was heard of two or more speedfreaks competitively injecting large amounts of methamphetamine. They would each mainline teaspoons of methamphetamine every hour or so. The winner was the one who could walk away. Whatever happened to the speedfreaks?

THE TOILET WATER FIX

One scene that remains etched in my memory occurred a dozen years ago at Piccadilly Circus, a favorite gathering place for London's heroin addicts. I was in the underground men's room when, through a partly opened door, I saw a young man filling a syringe with water from the toilet bowl. He had apparently obtained sterile syringes and sterile heroin from the nearby pharmacy, yet he preferred the water closet to the cleaner water from the nearby wash basins. I immediately realized why British addicts get hepatitis and other infections as frequently as their American counterparts who do not have access to sterile materials. This young man seemed to have a singular disregard for his well-being.

SMOKE GETS IN MY ARTERIES

Another much more distant memory that will not go away is of a patient who had just been admitted to the surgical service where I was an intern. He had an admitting diagnosis of Buerger's disease (an obliterative disease of the small and medium blood vessels related to heavy smoking) and had amputations, at various levels, of all four extremities. When I asked what brought him into the hospital, he replied with a particular intensity, "I'd like the surgeon to fix a skin flap on my right arm stump so that it will hold a cigarette."

THE 'GARBAGEHEAD'

A final reminiscence: during the 1960s, when the flower children began moving from the Haight-Ashbury to agrarian communes, I visited one in Northern California to try to understand the new phenomenon. This was a drug-using group that wanted to return to nature while living better through synthetic chemistry. One of the membership was referred to by the others as a "garbagehead."

He would consume any pill or liquid that came his way, known and unknown. He seemed to want only to get away from his ordinary consciousness. It didn't matter how or in which direction.

SUMMARY

Although an immediate survival drive does exist—except in the instance of suicide—a survival instinct that preserves the individual over the long term is not always clearly observable. Those who will shorten or interrupt their lives often are involved in the substance abuse scene, usually as high-dose, compulsive users. Not too much can be done to counteract the overriding need to use drugs perniciously. At the very least, users should be clearly informed of their limited outlook for survival so that ignorance is not a factor in their self-destruction.

The question, of course, is "Why?" Is their drug overuse an unextinguishable behavioral pattern that cannot be broken? Is it a countervailing death instinct? Is it depression or denial? Or is it, indeed, an inability or a refusal to behave as though a personal future existed? The answer remains obscure, but the same in-depth psychodynamic studies should be done with these people as have been performed on suicidal individuals.

26. Alcohol-Drug Combinations

Now that alcohol-containing beverages have become basic mood-altering substances upon which a variety of other drugs are overlaid, some consideration should be given to the implications and impacts of such multiple drug use.

The difficult problems of studying one drug are multiplied when two or more substances are used together, and definitive investigations in this area are not yet available. Some circumscribed work can be mentioned; the rest of our information on drug-alcohol combinations is derived from clinical impressions.

REASONS FOR ALCOHOL-DRUG USE

When drugs are taken together it is usually for one of four reasons.

1. Additional Drugs Are Used to Intensify the Effect of the Primary Substance

Since combining depressants are either additive or potentiating, they are frequently added to alcohol. When the marihuana or the heroin is weak, alcohol is added to reinforce the effects. When sleeping pills do not work, a quantity of ethanol is consumed along with them. If a few drinks don't seem to unwind the tense individuals, tranquilizers might be added.

2. Multiple Drugs May Be Used to Reduce the Undesirable Side Effects of the Primary Agent

Barbiturate-amphetamine combinations are popular because some people dislike the "wired up" feeling of large amounts of amphetamines. Alcohol has been employed by amphetamine abusers for similar purposes. In addition, they use large amounts of alcohol when coming down from an amphetamine binge to help induce sleep. Kipperman reports on a group of heavy drinkers who used moderate amounts of amphetamines to keep from passing out so that they could continue to drink. This practice could be hazardous because the built-in safeguard against overdosing with alcohol, namely unconsciousness, is evaded.

3. One or More Drugs May Be Used to Substitute for the Preferred Drug When It Is in Short Supply or Unavailable

When a heroin "panic" is on, narcotic addicts will drink large amounts of codeine cough syrup or alcohol, or swallow any available sedative. These drugs will not prevent all of the symptoms of the abstinence syndrome but they will keep the user relatively comfortable.

4. In Some Instances a Hodge-podge of Chemicals Is Taken Together without Particular Rationale or Interest in How They Will Interact

This is the "garbage head" syndrome, still occasionally seen among those who have little concern for their physical or mental health. It is difficult to understand the random ingestion of assorted psychochemicals. One suspects that the self-concept of such individuals must be quite low. The statement that they make with their omnivorous drug taking seems to be: "Anything is better than what I am."

EFFECTS OF ALCOHOL-DRUG USE

That alcohol taken in conjunction with other mind-altering drugs can be a serious matter is confirmed by the Drug Abuse Warning Network summaries. DAWN obtains reports from emergency rooms, crisis centers, and medical examiners in 24 urban areas on the frequency of drug mentions.

Alcohol alone is not included, but alcohol-in-combination with other drugs is. For the latest month available, April, 1977, alcohol-in-combination was the leading item in medical examiners' mentions. It was second in emergency room and crisis center mentions. Ethanol-sedative and ethanol-opiate combinations were the most frequent causes of death reported by medical examiners, exceeding deaths due to heroin alone.

SOME COMBINATIONS

If the use of alcohol and caffeine is set aside, the joint use of alcohol and tobacco is the most frequent combination. Heavy drinkers tend to be heavy smokers; in fact, in one survey, they smoked more than mental patients, drug addicts, and a normal control group. Objectively, there is little to recommend this combination. Performance is not improved as compared to alcohol alone, and some investigators have even found a decrement on performance tests. It must be that subjectively something satisfactory happens. An alternative explanation is that heavy smoking and drinking are conditioned behaviors and have little to do with feelings of satisfaction.

Now that some recent data indicates that cancers of the head, neck, and esophagus are more frequent in alcoholics who smoke excessively than in alcoholics who do not, or in heavy smokers who do not drink inordinately, this abuse combination assumes added importance. The speculation offered for the increased incidence of upper digestive tract cancers in this population is that alcohol may increase the solubility of the carcinogen in tobacco.

ALCOHOL AND SEDATIVE-HYPNOTICS

Many of the alcohol-sedative adverse interactions can happen in patients who drink only moderately, and are, by no means, limited to the chronic alcoholic. A fatality can occur at BAC (blood alcohol concentrations) of 0.1 mg percent 4–5 ounces of whiskey) combined with a blood barbiturate level of 0.5 mg percent of pentobarbital in a non-tolerant person. Ordinarily, the lowest level of blood barbiturate that can be associated with death is about 1.0–1.5 mg percent of hypnotic barbiturate. Much less alcohol and hypno-sedatives are also needed to produce severe states of intoxication.

This group contributes substantially to the "accidental suicide" by overdosing out of confusion, memory impairment or a lack of information about the synergistic effect of the depressant drugs. After a night of heavy drinking it may not be a good idea to take four or five sleeping pills in order to get a good night's rest. The rest may be unexpectedly long.

ALCOHOL AND MINOR TRANQUILIZERS

A lack of public awareness exists about the decremental effects of combined minor tranquilizers and alcohol on alertness and psychomotor skills. Benzo-diazepines may increase alcohol blood levels and add their depressant effect to those of moderate to large amounts of alcohol. Driving skills with meprobamate and alcohol are impaired over and above the drowsiness and inattention that occurs.

It is clear from the experimental studies of performance and from actual accident reports that have been studied utilizing blood testing for psychotropic drugs, that combinations of alcohol and the minor tranquilizers are more disruptive of driving and related behavior than either drug alone. Nor is the practice of driving under the influence of such a combination rare. Finkle's study showed that 10 percent of arrested drivers had both alcohol and a minor tranquilizer in their blood stream.

ALCOHOL AND OPIATES

This combination of consciousness-changing drugs is important for several reasons.

1. Patients on methadone maintenance are known to abuse alcohol; in fact, about a quarter of them have substantial problems with alcohol. The death rate of methadone maintenance patients who drink heavily is as much as 10 times as great as those methadone maintenance patients who abstain.

2. Both alcohol and heroin damage the liver. Heroin use introduces hepatitis B through contaminated injections. Alcohol excess induces alcoholic hepatitis and cirrhosis. The combination can lead to fulminating liver disease. More than 20 percent of New York City heroin addicts showed evidence of chronic alcoholism at autopsy.

3. The depressant effects of alcohol and opiates are additive, if not supra-additive, and this can be deadly. If a person has become addicted to both narcotics and alcohol, the treatment of withdrawal becomes much more complicated.

4. From studies of double addicted people, it seems that their prognosis for recovery is worse. They are a more disturbed and antisocial group, and their behavior is more aberrant.

ALCOHOL AND MARIHUANA

Although both of these drugs worsen performance, recent studies reveal that together an additional decrement in manual dexterity, vigilance, information processing, temporal organization, and perceptual control occurs. Pot and pop wines or beer have become a frequently used mixture. This particular combination also increases the heart rate to the point that people with borderline cardiac function may decompensate while under the influence.

ALCOHOL AND STIMULANTS

The common assumption that strong black coffee antagonizes the intoxicating effects of alcohol is not completely true. Caffeine does improve reaction time, but other tests of manual dexterity, mental arithmetic, perceptual speed, verbal fluency, etc., were either uninfluenced or were performed worse after caffeine. Caffeine also has no effect on the BAC. It is possible that a drinker may feel more alert after three cups of hot coffee (300 mg of caffeine) and will attempt to drive. But he will remain handicapped in many areas of psychomotor coordination, in search and recognition activities, and in other complex tasks.

Some mention has already been made of possible joint uses of amphetamines and alcohol. Cocaine and alcohol combinations are used in a similar fashion: to make the heavy drinker more alert and to help the cocaine user reduce the tension and edginess of that stimulant.

ALCOHOL AND OTHER DRUGS

Now that antidepressants such as amitriptyline (Elavil) and doxepin (Sinequan) are becoming abused drugs, the effects of their combination with alcohol should be noted. They potentiate the depressant effects of alcohol. Operating machinery or driving a car while under the influence of the combination may be hazardous. The effects of the major tranquilizers and the sedative antihistamines are enhanced by alcohol beverages in a similar manner. The over-the-counter sleeping potions contain scopolamine and an antihistamine. These drugs can lead to more CNS depression than expected when used with alcohol.

A common combination consists of the use of alcohol together with analgesics like aspirin. This joint use does not seem to lead to additional behavioral impairment. However, the effect of salicylates on the clotting mechanism, and the irritant effects of both substances on the stomach lining have caused gastric hemorrhages, some of which have been life-endangering.

Volatile solvent inhalers also are known to drink wine or beer while sniffing. Alcohol is chemically closely related to some solvents, and it adds to the anesthetizing effect of all of them.

DRIVING AND ALCOHOL-DRUG USE

The presumptive level of driving while intoxicated has been a BAC of 0.1 mg percent. Certain countries and states are looking into the adverse effects of lower BACs on driving performance, levels between 0.05 and 0.1 mg percent, and some are considering a lowering of the BAC presumptive of intoxication.

In a recent report from California as many as 22 percent of drivers who were stopped for driving under the influence had detectable marihuana or marihuana and alcohol levels. This is the first study of its kind because roadside testing for THC has only recently become available.

Combinations of alcohol with sedatives, tranquilizers, narcotics, antihistamines, and marihuana can only worsen driving performance because the depressant effects of the combinations are, at least, additive. Combinations of stimulants with alcohol may not improve the operation of a car. Although reaction time may be reduced, other, more complex functions necessary for the driving situation are either unchanged or less satisfactorily performed.

Even when drugs are used in therapeutic doses and not in the amounts taken by abusers, their joint use with alcohol can be hazardous. A Scandanavian study examined the blood levels of 74 drivers in accidents who required hospitalization for their injuries. They were compared with 204 drivers who were not in traffic accidents.

Of those hospitalized, 41.8 percent had measurable blood alcohol concentrations, 9.5 percent had detectable diazepam (Valium) levels, and 10.8 percent had both drugs in their bloodstream. The control group revealed that 1.5 percent had alcohol, 2 percent had diazepam, and none had both drugs on testing.

SUMMARY

We appear to have entered a second, more complicated, phase of drug abuse. Although pure alcoholics and addicts still can be found, the use of multiple drugs is becoming more frequent. In fact, it is becoming a sort of cottage industry to figure out new mixtures of chemicals and spread the word by means of the underground press.

We are witnessing a potpourri of drug-taking by barefoot psychopharmacologists whose trial and error chemical blends never have been tested for safety. The result has been a more precarious form of drug-taking than when single drugs were abused.

27. Pharmacology of Drugs of Abuse

This chapter is revised from a paper read at the International Conference on Drug Dependence, May 5-7, 1976, Rome, Italy.

Why are certain drugs abused? Why should one drug be preferred over another although both belong to the same pharmacologic class? What kinds of emotional experiences are sought by abusers of drugs?

All substances of abuse alter consciousness and mood. Consciousness is either raised or lowered. The varieties of changes in awareness range from a complete obliteration of consciousness, such as large doses of central nervous system (CNS) depressants can bring, to a vast intensification of awareness as experienced in the LSD state.

However, psychochemicals also exist that induce markedly altered states of awareness and yet they are never—or rarely—sought out for this purpose. No one seems to relish the diminution of consciousness that accompanies ingestion of the neuroleptics. The author has never met a chlorpromazine addict although he has read case reports of one or two. Street dealers do not stock the phenothiazines, the butyrophenones, or the thioxanthines. If they did, few of their customers would be interested. Why not? Perhaps because they have unpleasant side effects, but more important, because they do not produce euphoria.

Just because a drug has unpleasant properties does not mean that it will not be abused. Some may be deterred by a vile tasting or smelling concoction, or one which produces a gastrointestinal upheaval, but others will indulge. *Datura strammonium*, also known as Jimson Weed, is singularly unpleasant but it has a few devotees. Nutmeg and mace (*myristica fragrans*) are difficult to swallow in intoxicating doses but some manage it.

The fly agaric (*amanita muscaria*) has noxious autonomic effects, and the peyote cactus (*lophophora Williamsii*) is far from enjoyable going down or coming back up. Nevertheless, they are sought after. For that matter, the first cigar or the first injection of an opiate can be associated with considerable gastrointestinal turmoil but people persist and acquire tolerance to these side effects.

Another reason why one drug may be preferred over another, similar drug is its rapidity of action. Secobarbital is preferred to phenobarbital for that reason, and cocaine preferred to amphetamines. Rapid onset of euphoric action, the "rush," is also why the intravenous or inhaled route are preferred to oral intake.

EUPHORIA

The feeling tone called euphoria, or "high," is perennially sought after. This sense of physical and emotional well-being has been searched for since the ascent of man and woman. Almost every society has its culturally acceptable euphoriant. We even have accumulating evidence that other animal species are inclined to use agents that will intoxicate them.

The long search for euphoria has some puzzling aspects. Not only stimulants but depressants also evoke the condition called "high." Apparently, it is the distancing from harsh reality that counts—the reduction in ego controls and the feeling of being "stoned." Certain people seem to have no particular need to be other than sober, while others do. The search for euphoria is for many really a flight from dysphoria, or from what is more painful, aphoria.

It is difficult to describe euphoria. Its pharmacology is far from clearly understood. It is not only the elimination of physical and psychological pain. There is a positive aspect to it which may be described as a feeling of rightness with oneself and with existence.

The more intense euphoric states of elation and ecstasy resemble those in which a stimulation of the reward centers of the posterior hypothalamus has occurred. There are clusters of noradrenergic neurones, and their electrical stimulation or microinjections of norepineophrine produces similar intense emotions. It is likely that cocaine and large doses of amphetamines act over such mechanisms.

A second road to euphoria is via tension and drive reduction and the associated drowsy, reverie state. When feelings of psychic emptiness and hunger are relieved, when disturbing sexual drives are set aside, and when a relaxed quietude intervenes, this is experienced as euphoric. The narcotics, working over serotonergic mechanisms, elicit such responses.

The hypnosedatives, the anxiolytics, alcohol, and the volatile inhalants provide still another pathway to euphoria. These chemicals depress CNS function. First, they depress the inhibitory controls over affect and behavior, releasing mental functioning from its usual internal double-checking system. The monitors over mood and behavior are attenuated. This is felt as enjoyable and releasing by most people. In larger doses, the depression extends to other mental functions including memory, judgment, and rational thought. These impairments also may be experienced as euphoric.

TOLERANCE

Abusable drugs have other important pharmacologic properties. Tolerance and abstinence effects are often, but not invariably, observed (Table 27–1). Cocaine, for example, does not produce tolerance except in very high doses. A cocaine withdrawal syndrome been described only under similar high dose states. It is not precisely known why this should be so. Admittedly, it is quickly metabolized, and therefore has a brief duration of action. Perhaps, the rate of degradation of cocaine cannot be increased even with frequent administration, and metabolic tolerance cannot develop, except in enormous doses.

At the opposite end of the tolerance spectrum, as few as three or four daily doses of LSD will result in a complete refractoriness to a challenge dose of the drug. Responsiveness to LSD is regained after two or three days of abstinence. The alleged lack of tolerance or even the reverse tolerance to cannabis is simply due to the use of weak material. When large amounts of potent cannabis or THC are employed, tolerance will develop within a few days.

CROSS TOLERANCE

Cross tolerance between the sedative-hypnotics, the minor tranquilizers, alcohol, and the anesthetics has been generally recognized. This means that the organism tolerant to one of these agents is tolerant to all. It also means that detoxification can proceed with any member of any class of depressants for all others. This is cross dependence. Cross tolerance and cross dependence between all narcotics exists, and also between hallucinogens like LSD, mescaline, and psilocybin, but not to THC.

WITHDRAWAL

The phenomenon of withdrawal is similarly variable. Narcotic and sedative withdrawal syndromes can be intense, in fact, life endangering, when high quality material has been used frequently over long periods of time. Sudden stoppage of alcohol and sleeping pills in a tolerant person results in a dramatic series of neuropsychiatric events (Table 27–2). This is the depressant withdrawal syndrome and is readily distinguished from the narcotic withdrawal syndrome except when they occur in a person simultaneously.

The stimulant withdrawal syndrome, I am convinced, is worthy of that

Table 27-1
Some Pharmacologic Properties of Abused Drugs

Drug Class	Example	Euphoria	Psychological Dependence	Tolerance	Withdrawal Syndrome
Narcotics	Heroin	+ + +	+ + +	+ + +	+ + +
Sedatives	Barbiturates	+ +	+ + +	+ +	+ + +
Anesthetics	Alcohol	+ +	+ + +	+ +	+ + +
	Toluene	+	+ +	+	(+)
Anxiolytics	Diazepam	+ +	+ +	+	+
	Meprobamate	+ +	+ +	+	+
Hallucinogens	LSD	+ +	+	+ + +	−
	THC	+ +	+ +	+	(+)
Stimulants	Amphetamines	+ + +	+ + +	+ +	+
	Cocaine	+ + +	+ + +	+	+
Ganglionic Stimulants	Tobacco	(+)	+ + +	+ +	+

158

designation. The long period of sleep after discontinuing high dose amphetamine intake, the enormous intake of food, the profound, sometimes suicidal depression, fatigue, and generalized achiness—these constitute a fairly characteristic abstinence picture, which was identified by studying the "speedfreak crash" of a half dozen years ago.

Table 27-2
Withdrawal Syndromes

	Narcotic* Withdrawal	Depressant** Withdrawal	Stimulant*** Withdrawal
Piloerection	X		
Lacrimination	X		
Rhinorrhea	X		
Diarrhea	X		
Muscle Spasm	X		
Muscle Pain	X		X
Nausea, Vomiting	X	X	
Delirium, Hallucinations	X	X	
Convulsions	X	X	
Insomnia	X	X	
Sweating	X	X	
Tremors		X	
Psychic Depression			X
Hyperphagia			X
Hypersomnia			X

*opium derivatives and synthetic narcotics
**hypnotics, sedatives, anxiolytics, alcohol
***amphetamines, anorectics, cocaine

In general, the higher the level of tolerance, the more pronounced the severity of the untreated withdrawal effects. The exception to this is observed with convulsions. Seizures appear to depend more upon duration of administration of the drug than the level of tolerance that develops. Tolerance also develops more rapidly with successive re-exposures to the drug or to drugs of the same general class.

Hallucinogens, except for cannabis, do not produce withdrawal symptoms. Whether cannabis does induce a full-fledged withdrawal pattern remains a matter for discussion. Certainly nausea, anorexia, jitteriness, and insomnia are recorded after discontinuance of large amounts. Whether major symptoms of withdrawal-like convulsions or delirium can occur remains unlikely.

Although, clinically, withdrawal symptoms appear to subside after detoxification, and the patient may feel well, a number of physiological indices remain abnormal. In the instance of the detoxified narcotic-dependent person, slight elevations of body temperature, blood pressure, and respiratory rate can be measured. A slight dilation of pupils is detectable after months of abstinence. Still later, a secondary abstinence phase has been described in which the above signs are reversed.

Even after more than a year of abstinence, previously addicted laboratory animals and man react to a single injection of morphine aberrantly. Altered reactivity can be found in the computer-analyzed EEG, in an analysis of REM sleep after injection, and in accelerated tolerance development to subsequent doses of morphine. It is postulated by some investigators that these long-persisting effects play a role in late relapse. Certainly, conditioning factors, which develop during addiction and withdrawal, can be the basis for relapse before they are eventually extinguished.

DEPENDENCE

The question of psychological dependence is not a profound one intrinsic in some basic drug mechanism. Instead, it derives from the desire to reexperience the euphoric or stress-relieving effects of the drug. With respect to dependence on tobacco, the psychomotor conditioning plays an important part in the approach behavior. The ritual of smoking is anxiety reducing and reinforcing, and the pharmacologic effects of nicotine are, perhaps, less significant. No doubt the ritual of cannabis smoking also contributes to the desired effects of that plant.

Physical dependence is simply the buildup of tolerance, the withdrawal syndrome on sudden discontinuance, and the desire to avoid withdrawal sickness. The craving is as much a desire to avoid the symptoms of withdrawal as a desire to experience the "high." Narcotic addiction, for example, demands a "fix" every eight hours or less, otherwise early withdrawal effects are noticed. The same is true of alcohol dependence, with the morning shakiness and hangover representing early withdrawal reactions.

SUMMARY

Although drugs of abuse have certain pharmacologic similarities, they also manifest distinct differences. They all may produce euphoria, but euphoria is many things. Tolerance, a withdrawal syndrome, and psychological dependence often occur, but some of these agents do not produce these phenomena. Perhaps a culture would be best advised to seek out the safest euphoriant and teach its members to avoid all others.

28. The Volitional Disorders

It may be worthwhile to consider the disorders of volition—the conditions we bring upon ourselves. This chapter will deal only with those involving the intake of some substance, the consumatory volitional disorders.

It is a bit old fashioned to speak of volition, of free will, at a time when enormous forces seem to dominate our existence. But no matter how compelling these are, a measure of choice still seems to remain.

As these disorders are examined, they do not seem to arise from some defect of the will. No one decides: "I will become an alcoholic—or an addict—or obese." Ordinarily, these maladies emerge after a long series of minimal decisions such as "I'll have another drink," or "I'll get stoned," or "I'll have a piece of pie a la mode." No conscious choice was ever made. Instead, the person slipped unknowingly into a pattern of behavior that culminated in a disturbance of some consequence.

Rather, will power could be operational after the condition has become manifest, and it is evident that a life-threatening disorder exists. We must be aware, however, of the overriding difficulties that the overindulger will experience in trying to eliminate the habits of a lifetime.

To stop doing something that allayed psychic distress for decades, either pharmacologically or symbolically, is extremely difficult. The usual rewards of tension reduction, relaxation, or unconsciousness are no longer available. Aversive life experiences can no longer be dealt with by the usual means, however harmful they may have been. Even the psychomotor satisfactions of the habit—whether it be fixing, gorging, guzzling, or smoking—are gone.

Six consumatory volitional disorders will be discussed. Others exist but they are less frequently seen than the half dozen to be mentioned.

EXCESSIVE SMOKING OF TOBACCO

Smoking is one of the more difficult of the disorders of volition to understand. The substance is widely available, legal, and socially acceptable. Most adults are or have been smokers.

When cigarette users are asked why they persist despite the hazards involved, they are hard-pressed to describe the rewards of smoking. Some will mention feelings of relaxation, others mild stimulation, but many notice little or no mood alteration. It is a trivial reward when compared to the exaltation of cocaine, the vast alterations of consciousness that is LSD, the orgasmic pleasure of a good bag of heroin, or even the oblivion that sleeping pills or booze can bring. The joys of smoking can hardly be a significant reason for its perpetuation.

Instead, we should look at the ritual of smoking as being rewarding, and the reinforcement of repetitive oral-manual routines many thousands of times a year as the element that serves to fix and perpetuate the behavior. In addition, nicotine has been shown to produce a withdrawal syndrome in laboratory animals when its administration has been suddenly discontinued. This has been confirmed in humans whose pitiful tales of the abstinence effects are rather commonplace.

A few years ago the Synanon administration decided that a noxious practice like smoking should be abolished in Synanon houses. Most of the residents were people who successfully had kicked their heroin addictions cold turkey. But a number of these residents had to leave Synanon because they were unable to kick cigarettes. Some of the others felt that coming off heroin was less stressing. What does this mean? Apparently, the cigarette habit is so dependency-producing because of the social mimicking displays, cultural persuasion, personal gratifications, and some physiologic reinforcers that relapse is more frequent than remission.

Of all the volitional disorders, smoking is as dangerous as any. In fact, although there are those who rationalize the data and say that the final proof is not yet in, the statistical and experimental evidence is better than we will ever have for any of the other drugs called dangerous. Next to excessive drinking, it probably causes more morbidity and mortality than any other drug, including one named heroin. It is a major factor in development of lung and other cancers and chronic pulmonary disease like bronchitis and emphysema, and it contributes to a variety of cardiovascular and gastrointestinal problems.

Unfortunately, the earlier hopes of a reduction in smokers and smoking that arose during the late 1960s have been frustrated. More people are smoking more now than ever. In the United States more than 4,000 cigarettes a year are consumed for every adult person over 15.

OVEREATING

Obesity is common in affluent societies. A quarter of the population in this country is obese; that is, more than 20 percent are over their ideal weight. With increasing age, overweight conditions increase. Interestingly, even in non-affluent countries obesity is also present. This is probably a reflection of the high symbolic value placed on food and the high carbohydrate diet available, usually consisting of potatoes, bread, and other starches.

Juvenile obesity is usually due to genetic-metabolic factors, familial-cultural patterns that encourage overeating, evidences of emotional deprivation (such as separation from mother), and combinations of these. Eating habits learned early tend to continue into adult life. Adult obesity increases the severity and mortality from diseases like hypertension, arteriosclerosis, diabetes, gout, and cholecystitis.

Eating is a gratifying sensory experience. People who have little to enjoy in other aspects of daily living may overeat to achieve a measure of satisfaction with their existence.

The ingestion of food can also be anxiety-reducing; the feeling of "being full" is relaxing to child and adult alike. Depression is generally accompanied by anorexia and weight loss, but compulsive overeating is also seen, and the extreme hyperphagias are either depressive or psychotic equivalents.

In such studies done to examine the psychological characteristics of very adipose people, a rather common finding consisted of a lowered self-esteem. There was an expectation of personal failure and rejection. Their anger was turned inward upon themselves with depressive equivalents and self-inflicted injuries occurring at a higher rate than among the non-obese control groups.

Like many other volitional conditions, overeating is an exaggeration of a normal process. It might be assumed, therefore, that obesity should readily respond to treatment. This is not so. When evaluated over long periods of time, the conventional therapies are unsuccessful. What is needed, of course, is a thorough reeducation and a reduction in the emotional problems of the patient.

EXCESSIVE USE OF SUGAR

Every child knows that sweets are reward foods. The taste of sweetness is sought by members of all societies and even by other species, including the dog and the monkey. This almost universal craving has led to a vast production and refining of sugar, which is one of the few foods we eat that is virtually 100 percent pure. In fact, it is too pure, stripped of valuable nutrients in order to be snow white.

The association between sugar intake and childhood dental caries is well established, but we prefer to flouridate our water rather than reduce sucrose consumption. The stress of high loads of sugar over many years is presumed to contribute to adult-type diabetes by exhaustion of the islet cells of the pancreas.

A number of primitive cultures have been studied following the introduction of refined sugar into their diet. It has been found that when the per capita consumption per year rises to about 70 pounds, the incidence of diabetes approaches that of civilized societies such as England and the United States, whose use is more than 100 pounds per person each year. The sweet tooth also gives rise to obesity over time. Using the above statistic, about 600 to 700 calories a day are derived from sugars.

No one is going to take our refined sugar away. But those who use large quantities should be aware of some possible undesirable consequences, especially if they are overweight or have an abnormal glucose tolerance test.

EXCESSIVE DRINKING OF CAFFEINATED BEVERAGES

Coffee and tea have long been inveighed against, more so in bygone times when it was the drink of extremists who wanted to overthrow the establishments of the day. Coffee houses were seditious places where plots were brewed along with the coffee. Today it is the most innocent of beverages, and the 100 mg of caffeine a cup it contains is harmless—except for certain people. A collaborative heart study that looked into the effects of various drugs, alcohol, and beverages suggested that drinking more than six cups of coffee daily increased the risk of myocardial infarction. Tea drinking was less damaging because it contains half as much caffeine and also has some theophylline, which is a mild coronary vasodilator.

Probably more common than coronary artery effects are the psychic disturbances that consistent coffee drinking evokes in some people. Disturbed sleep is a well-known occurrence, but daytime irritability, nervousness, restlessness, and headache are not so uncommon. Some people describe withdrawal effects from caffeine, including impaired alertness, headache, and shakiness.

The drinking of caffeinated beverages is one of the more benign of the volitional disorders. It would be regrettable if that pleasure were eliminated. However, with the advent, at last, of potable decaffeinated coffees, those sensitive to the effects of the alkaloid can switch. Perhaps those who are double-digit coffee drinkers should do likewise.

VOLITIONAL DISORDERS ASSOCIATED WITH ABUSABLE DRUGS

The inordinate use of mind-altering drugs can be life-impairing and life-endangering. Almost all of these drugs, used in large amounts over prolonged periods, are hazardous to health by producing physical damage or some mental disorganization. What must be remembered is that drug abusers do not consciously want to shorten or terminate their lives. Some of them are self-treating their depression or their schizophrenic symptoms. Some are using drugs as a means of coping, however maladaptively, with stress. Some have little or no future orientation, no concept of tomorrow, and thus no need to be concerned about survival. Therefore, what we called risk taking may not be that to the risk taker. When we see a heroin addict looking for the "pusher" whose junk has just killed someone, he is merely looking for extra good stuff, not death.

The chronic lethal states will not be considered at this time. Instead, the focus will be on the acute disasters that can befall a chemically intoxicated individual.

Narcotics

The junkie is engaged in a high-risk occupation. He is apt to incur accidental or deliberate injury or death from many sources: muggers, his friends, his pusher, the police, and others. His suicide rate is 20 to 50 times that of the population at large. It is believed that each year 1 to 2 percent of the heroin addicts die from overdose or other acute reactions to the injected material. The numbers of street addicts over 60 are remarkably few. Some mature out—that is, give up heroin—but most will die before achieving that state.

Sedatives

Like the narcotic addict and the alcoholic, the habitual user of sleeping pills is accident prone and suicide prone. Barbiturates are now the second most popular means of suiciding, and they are first among the methods used by women. The "accidental suicide" has been well described by Kubie and others. This is the person who uses combinations of depressants in sufficient quantities to knock out the respiratory center. The most popular combination at the moment seems to be alcohol, a minor tranquilizer, and a barbiturate. The additive or potentiating effects of such polydrug use can result in death without any overt intent to do one's self in.

Stimulants

The heavy amphetamine user, as epitomized by the "speedfreak," is indeed a "death tempter" and "death defier" as described by Shneidman. Injecting gram quantities of amphetamines into one's vein can be devastating pharmacologically and behaviorally. The resulting combination of impulsivity, hyperactivity, and paranoid thinking can lead to all kinds of trouble. A half-dozen years ago something called "speed roulette" was still around. It consisted of two "freaks," each attempting to outdo the other in the amounts of "speed" they injected. The one who could not walk away lost.

Hallucinogens

Sudden death in connection with taking a drug like LSD is infrequent. When it occurs, it is usually due to a grandiose overestimate of one's powers. This results in attempts to fly or walk on water, all unsuccessful to date. Suicide is rare, and homicides even more so.

ALCOHOLISM AND ALCOHOL ABUSE

Alcoholism abounds with paradoxes. It is the most common and serious problem of all the drug dependencies, yet it is the most socially acceptable. While 95 percent of the adult drinkers apparently can drink without harming themselves, 5 percent are drinking destructively. It is not easy to predict who will become one of the 5 percenters. It is a malady in which the etiologic agent is obvious, but the prevention and cure elude us. One man's heavy social drinking is another's pathological dependence on alcohol.

Booze is ordinarily consumed to reduce anxiety, except that its chronic use increases anxiety levels. It is employed as a social lubricant to increase friendliness and good cheer, yet it is clearly the most violence producing of all drugs. And then, of course, the paradox of volition: why do millions impair their health, shorten their lives, disorganize their families and destroy themselves socially and financially by drinking excessively?

The story needs no retelling here about physical and mental damage, about the social and economic costs, about accidents, and the other prices paid by the 10 million alcohol abusers and 190 million nonabusers.

What we are interested in is: Why? Is it genetic predisposition, maladaptive response to environmental stress, permissive cultural attitudes, personality susceptibility, metabolic deficiency, or some malignant, learned behavior? The answer is: It's all of these in varying degrees in different individuals. And what of the will? Volition could overcome all of these factors, but extreme loading makes willful correction much more difficult.

Since the abuse of alcohol is so widespread and disastrous in its effects, perhaps a solution might be to replace the personal will with a political will. When a substance is so intermeshed into the social structure as alcohol, no government interdiction or prohibition can work. The only point to be made is that if alcohol were a newly discovered drug, and if it were submitted to the F.D.A. for marketing, it could hardly be approved for sale. The adverse effects and complications of extensive use are simply too many.

29. Symptoms and Signs of Drug Abuse

In this chapter the following definitions are used:
Depressants: *All narcotics, sedatives, tranquilizers, volatile solvents, alcohol.*
Narcotics or opiates: *Opium, heroin, morphine, Demerol, methadone, Dilaudid, codeine.*
Sedatives: *Barbiturate and non-barbiturate sedatives and hypnotics.*
Tranquilizers: *The minor tranquilizers such as meprobamate and chlordiazepoxide.*
Stimulants: *Amphetamines, cocaine, Ritalin, Preludin.*
Hallucinogens: *LSD, mescaline, DMT, MDA Sernyl, psylocybin.*

The widespread misuse of drugs makes it necessary to consider this condition in the differential diagnosis of a wide variety of medical, surgical, and psychiatric illnesses. This is particularly true in adolescent medicine, but adults are by no means excluded from the untoward effects of mind-altering drugs. The more common symptoms and signs that are encountered will be reviewed by system.

ASSOCIATED CONDITIONS

A number of ailments that occur more frequently in heavy drug users than in the population at large are mentioned here. They are not the result of drug ingestion; they are due to the life-style of the "head," particularly when he congregates in urban ghettos or in unsanitary communes.

Poor hygiene and a lowered resistance to infection produce an increased incidence of upper respiratory infections, trench mouth, scabies, pediculosis, and impetigo. Poorly healing sores are frequently seen. Dietary faddism may induce mineral, vitamin, or protein deficiencies. Dental caries is one of the frequent reasons for visits to free clinics and other emergency health facilities. Lacerations of the soles of the feet are occupational hazards for the unshod. Streptococcal sore throat, viral hepatitis, mononucleosis, tuberculosis, and leptospirosis, along with other infections including the childhood contagious diseases, are present in greater than average community levels because of malnutrition, crowding, dirt, or neglect. Food poisoning epidemics from poorly prepared or improperly stored food or contaminated water have occurred during a few rock festivals.

Ringworm, seborrhea, and jock itch are well known. The incidence of acne is high even for this age group. Whether this is the result of poor skin care is uncertain. Some investigators believe that marihuana can exacerbate acne.

Because of casual attitudes toward the variety of sexual activities, syphilis, gonorrhea, and other veneral diseases are increasing in the population. The chancre may sometimes be found in extragenital sites such as the lip, tonsil, finger, or nipple. Nonspecific urethritis and cervicitis, trichomoniasis, and moniliasis are also prevalent. Hemorrhoids and anal fissures in male or female youngsters may be a complication of unusual sex practices.

With the increased violence that has come to the scene, the results of beatings, shootings, and stabbings have required treatment. Only a minority of these assaults have been due to drug-induced aggressiveness. Usually they are the result of the intervention of criminal or psychopathic elements into a colony of innocents who are unable to cope with them.

GENERAL SYMPTOMS

Weight loss or malnutrition can accompany chronic, heavy use of most drugs. Amphetamines and cocaine have a direct effect upon the satiety centers producing anorexia. The heroin addict, in addition to a reduced appetite, tends to use money for drugs, not food. Exhaustion is the end state of ''speed'' runs and other extended drug binges. Impotence and amenorrhea are reflections of a general drug-induced debility, with depressant drugs further dampening libido and hormonal function.

Fever is found when stimulants or hallucinogens increase sympathetic tone and the metabolic rate. It is also present during the depressant withdrawal period. Needle-borne infections, of course, will also produce elevated temperatures.

SKIN

Color Changes

Jaundice is often noted when the patient has serum or viral hepatitis. Cyanosis is maximal in opiate overdose, but can also be present in sedative overdoses and during convulsive episodes. LSD produces a flush during its period of action. The discoloration of the fingers in heavy cannabis smokers differs in location from tobacco stain. In the "pothead" it is on the thumb and forefinger, in the tobacco smoker it is on the fore and middle finger.

The "tracks" of long-standing opiate and, less frequently, long-term barbiturate and amphetamine "mainliners" are pigmented, linear markings along the course of superficial veins of the arms, legs, and penis. They are caused by injected foreign particles or low-grade infections. Since they last indefinitely, efforts are sometimes made to cover them with a tatoo. Long sleeved clothing is worn during warm weather for similar reasons. The puncture needle marks can be detected for only a few days or a week unless an inflammatory reaction has occurred. Thrombophlebitis of the veins is occasionally seen and is the result of injecting irritating or infectious material. Abscesses or depressed, scarred areas are present in "skin poppers," particularly when the opiate injection has been made into the fatty tissue of the upper arm or thigh.

Other Skin Changes

Ankle edema can be found in an occasional patient on methadone maintenance. Gooseflesh is a reliable, objective sign of withdrawal from opiates. Sweating is prominent during the withdrawal states and during high dose amphetamine use. Patients on methadone maintenance may complain of it. Almost any drug can cause a rash. Barbiturate and tranquilizer rashes are quite common. The pustular rash of chronic bromidism should be recalled. Acne rosacea and dilated facial venules accompany heavy alcohol intake. Solvent inhalers may present with a rash around the mouth and nose.

EYE, NOSE, AND THROAT

Eye

The conjunctivitis (red eye) of the cannabis user and the alcoholic is well known. Dilated pupils are encountered during hallucinogenic, volatile solvent, or stimulant exposure. Anticholinergic drugs like belladonna, henbane, or Jimson weed will also dilate the pupils. Constricted pupils are the hallmark of opiate activity. During withdrawal or following Nalline injection they will dilate. Solvents will cause tearing, and lacrimation is also a part of the opiate withdrawal state.

Nose

Runny nose occurs during the opiate abstinence syndrome. Septal ulceration in connection with cocaine and amphetamine "snorting" is documented. The intense vasoconstriction from cocaine can cause a septal perforation.

The odor of some misused items can be detected during and after use. Volatile solvents and alcohol are partially excreted via the respiratory tract;

therefore they can be smelled for an hour or more after intake. The odor of marihuana smoke resembles burnt rope and is perceptible in the exhaled breath, the clothing, or the room for a while. Incense may be used to disguise the odor.

Throat

Uvular edema is described following heavy bouts of hashish smoking. Users of marihuana, anticholinergic compounds, amphetamines, and opiates may complain of dryness of the mouth. Sernyl (phencyclidine) is said to cause salivation. Laryngeal spasm and freezing occur when aerosol sprays are inhaled rapidly for purposes of intoxication.

RESPIRATORY

Bronchitis is a symptom in those who persistently smoke such irritating substances as tobacco, marihuana, and hashish. Bronchial carcinoma and emphysema have not yet been demonstrated to be related to cannabis use, as they have to tobacco. Asthmatic attacks have been precipitated by LSD and cannabis in predisposed individuals. Aspiration pneumonia can take place during a coma due to depressant drugs. Pneumonia, pulmonary abscesses, embolism, and fibrosis all may develop in connection with injection of insoluble or septic materials into a vein. Talc emboli occur after Ritalin, Pyribenzamine, or other talc base tablets are dissolved and injected.

Apnea is a manifestation of depressant poisoning. Acute pulmonary edema is the common cause of death in opiate overdose. It is associated with right ventricular dilation, hypotension, hyperpnea, and cyanosis. Hyperpnea is a possible sequel to high amphetamine doses. Chest pain is also a component of the amphetamine overdose picture.

Instances of suffocation are known in which glue sniffers fell unconscious on the rag containing the material. Other cases have occurred when volatile solvents were sniffed in closed spaces—for example, a plastic garment bag.

CARDIOVASCULAR

Endocarditis of bacterial or fungal origin is a recognized complication of unsterile intravenous injections. Cardiac arrhythmias are associated with amphetamine overdose. This condition, also called "overramped," is manifested by tachycardia and hypertension. Other reasons for a rapid pulse are cannabis, hallucinogen, or cocaine use. During opiate withdrawal the pulse rate is often rapid. Sino-atrial or A-V arrest is precipitated by the Freon sprays in the presence of hypoxia.

Cerebral hemorrhages in young people may be caused by dramatic elevations of blood pressure due to amphetamine injections. Bradycardia and hypotension are concomitants of opiate overdose. Shock is a development in serious poisoning due to narcotics or sedatives. An angiitis of small and medium calibre arteries has been reported after prolonged amphetamine use, particularly in high doses.

GASTROINTESTINAL

Nausea and vomiting accompany the ingestion of many drugs. This is particularly true of peyote. The first few injections of opiates may produce vomiting, but tolerance to this effect is rapidly acquired. Loss of appetite is noteworthy when stimulants are used. It is also routinely present during the LSD state. On the other hand, hyperphagia is remarked upon by about half of cannabis users. A ravenous appetite is also present during amphetamine withdrawal. Opiate users are usually constipated, with diarrhea and abdominal cramps occurring during withdrawal. Diarrhea is experienced by some cannabis users. In folk medicine it has been used in the treatment of constipation. Complaints of abdominal pain have been heard from an occasional amphetamine abuser and during opiate withdrawal. Sometimes the pain is severe enough to cause one to consider it a surgical emergency.

Hepatitis as a disease of the unsterile needle or of the life style of the "head" needs no additional comment. Large amounts of amphetamines and alcohol have a hepatotoxic capability. The role of malnutrition and hypovitaminosis in liver damage due to these two drugs is acknowledged. Liver damage due to volatile solvents, particularly carbon tetrachloride, is known.

HEMATOPOIETIC

Case reports of aplastic anemia due to benzene inhalation are in the literature. Nutritional anemias are found whenever intense preoccupation with mind-altering drugs occur. Malaria is not encountered as frequently as in the past in connection with the use of group syringes and needles. Blood stream infections are always a possibility under such circumstances. Bleeding tendencies are a real possibility in heavy drinkers due to their varicosities and prothrombin deficiency.

MUSCULOSKELETAL

Serious musculoskeletal disorders do not play a noteworthy role in drug abuse problems. Muscle wasting as a part of the severe weight loss in "speedfreaks" is seen. Tremors are a common symptom during hallucinogen and stimulant use. In chronic alcohol, sedative, and opiate users the tremor may persist after the drugs are no longer used. During opiate withdrawal muscle cramps and spasms can cause considerable discomfort. The muscle jerks may involve an entire extremity (kicking the habit). The aches and pains of all withdrawal states are referred to the muscles and bones.

NEUROLOGICAL

The hallucinogens and stimulants increase and quicken the deep tendon reflexes. The opposite is true of the sedatives and narcotics. Headache is complained of during amyl nitrite inhalation. Occasional marihuana users will speak of a hangover headache. The prototypical symptom of the hung-over drinker or solvent sniffer is headache.

The stimulants and hallucinogens produce insomnia. Sedatives, cannabis, tranquilizers, and narcotics induce drowsiness. The depressant drugs can result in stupor or in coma. This includes the anesthetics, such as nitrous oxide, the aerosols, and volatile solvents. Convulsions are infrequently observed during LSD and amphetamine use. They constitute a part of the abstinence syndrome for all depressant drugs. Hyperactivity is associated with the amphetamines and cocaine. Stereotyped activity is also characteristic of these drugs. Repetitive, useless activities of a simple nature such as picking the skin, pacing, or stringing and unstringing beads might be continued for hours. A cerebellar syndrome consisting of ataxia, nystagmus, diplopia, clumsiness, and slurred speech is associated with depressant intoxication.

Some of the disease entities seen in connection with drug abuse include peripheral neuritis, Korsakoff's and Wernicke's syndromes (alcohol), tetanus, and encephalitis (needle-borne infection). A case of lead encephalopathy due to gasoline sniffing has been reported. A single report of cerebral atrophy in chronic cannabis users has not been confirmed.

PSYCHIATRIC

Some of the signs of involvement in the drug life include behavioral toxicity; that is, behavior becomes destructive to the individual or those around him. Changes from previous behavior patterns occur: changes in the sleep-wake cycle, changes in choice of friends and associates, changes in mood including unpredictability and impulsivity, changes in the direction of decreased school or work performance, and changes in truthfulness and honesty. Other changes observed are in goal-directedness, drives, and attitudes. This is the amotivational syndrome. These alterations are not diagnostic of drug abuse, but that condition ought to be considered when they become obvious.

During cannabis, stimulant, and hallucinogen trips panic and anxiety states can prevail. An acute psychotic or paranoid reaction may intervene. A toxic delirium is possible with every drug that has been used for its mind altering properties. Deliria are also characteristics of the depressant abstinence syndromes, with confusion, hallucinations, and delusions regularly seen. It is said that certain drugs have specific hallucinatory qualities. For example, cocaine is supposed to provide tactile hallucinations usually of insects in or on the skin. Folk beliefs allege that alcoholic deliria consist of seeing strange animals such as pink elephants. These tales are often mistaken. Alcohol can induce an acute auditory hallucinosis during which the individual is quite well oriented except that he hears voices, music, or other sounds that are not present. Depressions may develop during LSD experiences, but are seen more often following that event. Particularly during the withdrawal phase following a binge of high dose amphetamines can the depression be profound. The suicide rate among all drug-dependent persons is high both during the intoxication and during the drug-free interval. Homicides may be more frequent with amphetamine in large doses than any other drug. Accidental death due to miscalculation of the environment is a possibility with every agent. Prolonged psychotic breaks are well known with the hallucinogens, the stimulants, alcohol, and the sedatives. Clinicians have diagnosed chronic brain syndromes in people who have taken LSD, PCP, amphetamines, and depressants over a long period of time.

CONCLUSION

Almost any organ system may be involved in the side effects of drug misuse. The possibility that presenting symptoms might be caused by drug exposure is worth entertaining. Occasionally, a perplexing diagnostic problem will be clarified when a detailed licit and illicit drug history is taken.

BIBLIOGRAPHY

General
- Cherubin, C. E. Acute addictive states. N.Y. State J. Med. 71:2391-2394 (Oct 14) 1971.
- Louria, D. B. Medical complications of drug abuse. Drug Therapy. (Aug) 1972, pp. 35-44.
- Lundberg, G. D. Complications of drug abuse. Calif. Med. 114: 77-78, 1971.

Amphetamines
- Kramer, J. C., Fischman, V. S. and Littlefield, D. C. Amphetamine abuse. JAMA 201:305-309 (July 31) 1967.

- Lynn, E. J. Amphetamine abuse. A "speed" trap. Psychiat. Quarterly 45:92–101, 1974.
- Margolis, M. T. and Newton, T. H. Methamphetamine (speed) arteritis. Neuroradiology 2:179–182, 1971.
- Tinklenberg, J. R. A clinical view of the amphetamines. Family Physician 4:81–86 (Nov) 1971.

Barbiturates

- Deveniji, P. and Wilson, M. Abuse of barbiturates in an alcoholic population. Canad. Med. J. Assn. 104:219–221, 1971.
- Norton, P. R. E. Some endocrinological aspects of barbiturate dependence. Brit. J. Pharmacol. 41:317–330, 1971.
- Shubin, H. and Weil, M. H. Shock associated with barbiturate intoxication. JAMA 215:263–268, 1971.
- Smith, D. E. and Wesson, D. R. A new method of treatment of barbiturate dependence. JAMA 213:294 (July 13) 1970.

Hallucinogens

- Bakker, C. B. The clinical picture in hallucinogen intoxication. Hospital Medicine. (Nov) 1969, pp. 102–114.
- Cohen, S. A classification of LSD reactions. Psychosomatics 12, 182–186, 1966.
- Frosch, W. A. The abuse of psychotomimetic drugs. Int. J. Addictions. 6:299–308 (June) 1971.
- Malleson, N. Acute adverse reactions to LSD in clinical and experimental use in the United Kingdom. Brit. J. Psychiat. 118:229–230, 1971.
- Schwartz, C. J. The complications of LSD: A review of the literature. J. Nerv. Ment. Dis. 146:174, 1968.
- Stern, M. and Robbins, E. S. Clinical diagnosis and treatment of psychiatric disorders subsequent to use of psychedelic drugs. In, *Psychedelic Drugs*, Grune & Stratton, New York, 1969.
- Taylor, R. L., Maurer, J. I. and Tinklenberg, J. R. Management of "bad trips" in an evolving, drug scene. JAMA 213:422 (July 20) 1970.

Marihuana

- Campbell, A. M. G., Evans, M., Thomson, J. L. G. and Williams, M. J. Cerebral atrophy in young cannabis smokers. Lancet 2(7736) 1219–1224 (Dec 4) 1971.
- Clark, L. D., Hughes, R. and Nakashima, E. N. Behavioral effects of marihuana. Arch. Gen. Psychiat. 23:193 (Sept) 1970.
- Keup, W. Psychotic symptoms due to cannabis abuse. Dis. Nerv. Syst. 31:119 (Feb) 1970.
- Kolansky, H. and Moore, W. T. Effects of marihuana on adolescents and young adults. JAMA 216, 486 (Apr 19) 1971.
- Talbott, J. A. Marihuana psychosis. JAMA 210:299, 1969.

- Tennant, F. S., Preble, M., Pendergast, T. S. and Ventry, P. Medical manifestations associated with hashish. JAMA 216:1965 (June 21) 1971.
- Weil, A. T. Adverse reactions to marihuana. N. E. J. Med. 282:907 (Apr 30) 1970.

Narcotics

- Cherubin, C. E. Infectious disease problem of narcotic addicts. Arch. Int. Med. 128:309–314 (Aug) 1971.
- Dole, V. P., Foldes, F. F., Trigg, H., Robinson, J. W. and Blatman, S. Methadone poisoning. N. Y. State J. Med. 71:541–543, 1971.
- Saylor, L. F. Induced vivax malaria among users of intravenous heroin. Calif. Med. 114:73–75, 1971.
- Stone, M. L., Salerno, L. J., Green, M. and Zelson, C. Narcotic addiction in pregnancy. Amer. J. Obstet. & Gynec. 109:716–723, 1971.
- Tartakow, I. J. Narcotic induced hepatitis. Amer. J. Med. 50:313–316, 1971.

Volatile Solvents

- Bass, M. Sudden sniffing death. JAMA 212:2075, 1970.
- Chapel, J. L. and Thomas, G. Aerosol inhalation for kicks. Missouri Med. 67:378, 1970.
- Press, E. and Done, A. K. Physiologic effects and community control measures for intoxication from the intentional inhalation of organic solvents I. Pediatrics 39:451, 1967. II. Pediatrics 39:611, 1967.
- Taylor, G. J. and Harris, W. S. Cardiac toxicity of aerosol propellants. JAMA. 214:81, 1970.

30. Skin Signs of Substance Abuse

The skin is almost all that we see of a person and it can be very revealing.

A glance at the skin may be rewarding for a clinician seeking diagnostic support in an obscure instance of some chemical dependency, or for an emergency room physician trying to understand why the patient is comatose, hardly breathing, and without a perceptible pulse.

ACUTE ALCOHOLIC INTOXICATION

Direct Signs of Drinking

The vasodilating effect of alcohol often produces a *flush*. Certain hypersensitive Asians and Eastern Europeans will flush strongly about the head and neck after ingesting very small quantities of alcoholic beverages. Drinkers who are receiving one of the antidiabetic sulfonamides tend to flush readily.

Naturally, anyone who takes a drink after swallowing Antabuse would show an intense red skin color in addition to the other symptoms of the alcohol-Antabuse reaction. The severe erythemas are thought to be caused by a sensitization to acetaldehyde. Since Antabuse inhibits the breakdown of acetaldehyde by interfering with the action of aldehyde dehydrogenase, the flush in that instance is almost certainly due to a high acetaldehyde blood level. *Red eye* is a suffusion of the conjunctiva associated with a prolonged bout of drinking.

Indirect Signs of Drinking

The clumsiness and the stuporous condition of the intoxicated person results in a number of cutaneous stigmata. *Cigarette burns* between the fingers and over the upper body are well known. Falls may result in *bruises* or *bleeding*.

Pressure ulcers over the bony prominences reflect long periods of immobility due to unconsciousness. In the south, drinkers who fall asleep out-of-doors may awaken with disseminated *fire ant stings*, while those who do the same in northern states in winter will develop *frostbite*, to say the least.

CHRONIC ALCOHOLISM

Direct effects

Jaundice may be seen in patients with either alcoholic hepatitis or cirrhosis. *Spider angiomata* and *telangiectases* are distributed over the upper thorax, neck, and head in steady drinkers.

The *caput Medusae* is a dilated, tortuous collection of veins surrounding the umbilicus in some cases in portal vein obstruction. It represents an attempt to form collateral pathways for the return of blood from the abdominal organs bypassing the scarred and occluded portal system in the liver. The phrase refers back to the head of Medusa, a mythological woman whose hair was turned into a mass of writhing snakes by Athena. Whoever looked at her was turned into stone.

Palmar erythema is a common sequel to heavy drinking. The syndrome of male *gynecomastia*, and sparse *chest, pubic*, and *axillary hair* is due to a toxic effect of alcohol on testicular hormone production.

Bleeding tendencies due to prothrombin deficiencies result in *purpura, nose* and *gum bleeds*, and other hemorrhagic displays. The *melanosis* seen in some cirrhotics might be caused by an associated pellagra. Alcoholic beriberi presents with a *scaly dermatitis* and *glossitis*. Cirrhosis is associated with *flat, opaque nails* with white transverse bands and tendency to develop *Dupuytren's contracture*. The nail fold is thinned and the cuticle is widened. About 10 percent of cirrhotics show *clubbing* of the fingers. *Erythematous skin nodules*, particularly on the legs, sometimes can be found. These are necrotic fat clumps secondary to the high lipase levels associated with pancreatitis.

Some skin diseases are caused by consistent heavy drinking, others are made worse by such indulgence. The nasal area can be involved with *acne rosacea* and *rhinophyma*. *Seborrhea* is common, and *nummular eczema* and *psoriasis* may be exacerbated. *Leukoplakias* are detectable on the oral mucous membranes, and a *black hairy tongue* or a green, *chlorophyl-stained tongue* are sometimes visible.

Indirect Signs

The life style of the Skid Row type of chronic drinker makes him liable to develop a number of cutaneous changes. Personal hygiene is neglected, and the dermatoses of improper diet and infection become apparent. *Sores* and *ulcerations* of the extremities, *scabies, pediculi* of the hair parts, and folliculitis of the bearded areas are seen. *Abscesses,* even *carbuncles,* are more frequent in this group than in the general population. *Tooth decay* and *gum boils* are common.

NON-MEDICAL NEEDLE USE AND SKIN SIGNS

Opiates, and in particular, heroin, are the most commonly injected drugs for non-medical purposes. However, amphetamines, cocaine, sedative-hypnotics, and an array of other substances are also injected subcutaneously, intramuscularly, or intravenously. The possible intravenous injection sites are numerous. After the veins of the arm are "buggered," those of hands, fingers, legs, neck, penis, and sublingual veins have been used.

Needle puncture marks may be identified for up to a week. They can be found over any accessible skin area, usually over the superficial veins. They should be looked for before punctures for medical purposes are begun. *"Pop"* *abscesses, ulcers,* and *scars,* the results of skin "popping," are visible over the upper arm, back, abdomen and thigh.

The toxic effect of quinine, often used as an adulterant for heroin, causes a necrotic breakdown of fat and skin. *Tracks* are linear, discolored, brownish streaks found along the course of subcutaneous veins. They are the result of unsterile injections along with deposition of particulate materials. They can last for years and become lighter as they age. Attempts to obliterate tracks by *bleaching* or *tattooing* have been made. *Thrombophlebitis* is a common finding that is associated with less-than-sterile punctures of the veins.

Two other cutaneous infections occur much less frequently: *camptodactylia* (edema and fibrosis of the fingers preventing their flexion) and *sphaceloderma* (necrosis of the skin).

"Shooting tattoos" are black spots caused by the carbon from a flamed needle being repeatedly injected under the skin. *Tourniquet discolorations* are circular markings where belts or ropes were repeatedly applied to occlude veins prior to injection. They represent cutaneous bleedings and pressure pigmentations of poorly fitting tourniquets applied over years. A mistaken intra-arterial injection can lead to *pain, swelling, cyanosis,* and *gangrene* of the extremity. Injecting barbiturates and related substances outside the vein can give rise to a woody cellulitis that is painful and inflamed. *Jaundice,* as one symptom of hepatitis, is often transmitted by the group use of infected needles.

SKIN MANIFESTATIONS OF THE ADDICTED LIFE STYLE

When existence centers around a chemical, many common health-sustaining practices are neglected. Skin and oral care are seldom practiced, and *trench mouth, skin infestations,* and *caries* are likely. *Linear, transverse scars* across the wrists are occasionally seen, the residuals of some unsuccessful suicide attempt in a person whose character structure and life style contribute to a depressive state. Dirt and infestations also result in *scratch excoriations*. Cigarette and match *burns* result from "nodding" while under the influence of heroin or sleeping pills. *Tattoos* indicating adherence to some deviant group or a deviant life style might be encountered. These are sometimes homemade. *Acanthosis nigricans* is sometimes seen in the armpits and may be related to inadequate hygiene or poor nutrition. The dermal consequences of avitaminosis, including *peleche*, have been observed. *Scabies* and *pediculosis* are found under conditions of inattention to cleanliness.

SKIN MANIFESTATIONS OF NARCOTIC USE

Opiate overdose is characterized by *pinpoint pupils, cyanosis, apnea*, and *coma*. As an exception, the pupils may be *dilated* when meperidine (Demerol) has been used. Terminally, extreme anoxia may cause constricted pupils, due to opiate overdose, to become dilated. During withdrawal from heroin and related drugs the pupils are usually dilated.

The potpourri of materials that go into the bag of heroin make allergic reactions a good possibility. A *fixed drug eruption* at the injection site, *urticaria*, and *purpura* have been recorded. The hives are the result of a histamine reaction and are supposed to be common when morphine is injected intravenously. These lesions may be *pruritic*, and *scratch marks* may be seen. *Piloerection* represents a valuable objective sign of narcotic withdrawal. An occasional patient on methadone maintenance will have *ankle edema*. *Sweating* is also a complaint of methadone maintenance patients.

COCAINE SKIN REACTIONS

The sniffing of cocaine can lead to *redness, ulceration*, and more rarely, *perforation* of the nasal septum. Cocaine has a vasoconstricting effect that impairs nutrition to the mucous membranes and, over time, causes necrosis. The paresthesias reported by cocaine users may account for the hallucinated "coke bugs." These imaginary insects, crawling under or on the skin, produce itching and can result in considerable *scratch marks*, sometimes with secondary infections.

SKIN CHANGES WITH OTHER DRUGS

During the period of LSD activity, the face is *flushed*. *Sweating* accompanies high-dose amphetamine use. Allergic rashes to barbiturates and other sedative-tranquilizer drugs occur from time to time. They may be *erythematous, pur-*

puric, or *urticarial.* Barbiturate or other sedative-hypnotic overdose is accompanied by either *contracted* or *unchanged pupil* size.

On the other hand, in glutethimide (Doriden) overdose, the *pupils* are *dilated* or *anisocoric.* *Bullae* on the dependent and pressure-bearing surfaces of the skin might be encountered in any deeply comatose patient. It is believed, however, that barbiturates adversely affect epidermal metabolism, and the sweat glands excrete a certain amount of barbiturates. Therefore, blisters may form more readily in the person unconscious from barbiturates.

Solvent inhalers may present with a *dermatitis* around the nose and mouth. Those who inhale spray paints may appear in an emergency room with the metallic silver or gold pigment on their face.

Gynecomastia in males who use marihuana chronically has been described, but it is a rarity. *Discolorations* of the fingers due to the marihuana tars might be seen between the thumb and index finger in heavy smokers who do not use a holder. A *conjunctivitis* is regularly seen during the period of marihuana use. An association between cannabis use and *acne* has been suggested. Chronic bromide use is associated with an *acneiform* or a *pustular eruption.*

SUMMARY

The skin is a revealing organ, and it can be helpful in clarifying some puzzling clinical problems. Most illicit drugs or their mode of use will produce cutaneous signs that can assist in the diagnostic process.

BIBLIOGRAPHY

- Committee on Alcoholism and Drug Dependence, A.M.A. *Medical Complications of Alcohol Abuse*, 1973.
- Korn, L. and Weidman, A. I. Pathogenesis and age of skin stigmata of narcotic addiction. *J.A.M.A.* 224:1433, 1973.
- National Drug Abuse Training Center, Medical Monograph Series, Vol. 1, No. 1, *Diagnosis and Evaluation of the Drug Abusing Patient*, Nov., 1976.
- Richter, R. W. *Medical Aspects of Drug Abuse.* Harper & Row, Hagerstown, MD, 1975.
- Young, A.W. et al. Skin stigmata of adolescent drug addiction. *Modern Treatment.* 9:117, 1972.

31. Geriatric Drug Abuse

The attention of the public and of the experts has been focused upon the youthful drug abuser. In fact, when we think about the addict or the drug-dependent person, it is the young "junkie" or "head" who comes to mind. A significant drug abuse problem also exists among the elderly. This is, in part, what the National Commission on Marihuana and Drug Abuse called "America's hidden drug problem." It is certainly more covert, less investigated, and less written about, but in certain respects it is just as worthy of serious study as the adolescent situation. The youngest may freak out in public places on alien psychochemicals. Meanwhile, the aged alcohol or drug abuser passes out quietly in his drab, furnished room or in some Skid Row alley.

The drugs of geriatric abuse are almost invariably depressants. Juveniles may seek an intensification of sensation and increased awareness from hallucinogens or stimulants although they, too, prefer "downers" these days. The use of central nervous system sedatives, hypnotics, alcohol, and tranquilizers are more and more the preferred mode of altering consciousness. When stimulants are misused by oldsters, it is in combination with sedatives or narcotics. Withdrawal from a frustrating existence and evasion of life stress is what is sought after rather than new experiences of hyperalertness.

One impressive observation is the great variability in the response of an old person to various amounts of a consciousness-changing drug. They may be hypersensitive to even average amounts of a psychochemical, barbiturates, for example. This is probably due to problems with detoxification and excretion. An impaired renal clearance or a reduced capacity to induce enzyme formation to detoxify a drug are conditions associated with the aging process. These physiologic impairments are associated with a psychological brittleness, which can produce mental confusion or a fluctuating delirium from ordinary quantities of a depressant. When recent memory and time orientation are adversely affected, supervision in the taking of prescribed drugs is needed. Otherwise, too much or too little will be self-administered.

THE NARCOTIC ADDICT

Aged opiate addicts can be sorted into at least two subgroups: surviving street addicts and medical addicts. A third group, probably disappearing, is the so-called Southern-type addict.

Street Addicts

Street addicts over 60 are not often seen. Before reaching that age most have either died from the consequences of injecting unsterile materials for decades, of overdosing, or they have been done in by the addict-associated diseases or trauma. A number tire out and no longer can keep up with their rigorous "junkie" careers of "hustling" and "copping." This phenomenon has been called "maturing out" of the drug scene. Just what the elements involved in "maturing out" consist of are not well understood. It does not appear to be a psychological maturation process in most instances, rather it is a matter of physical exhaustion.

It takes a combination of an excellent constitution, extraordinary good luck, and an unusual survival ability to manage to celebrate one's 60th birthday as a street addict. By that time the old junkie has learned how to remain invisible. In order to avoid police harrassment and the neighborhood rip-off artists, he maintains the lowest of profiles. His criminal activities decrease. His lack of satisfaction with street heroin may convert him to a user of methadone, morphine, Dilaudid, or Demerol. These can be bought on the street or "conned" out of well-meaning doctors. If things get too rough he will "shoot" paregoric or drink codeine cough syrup by the four ounce bottle where these items are still available without a prescription.

Some over-sixty addicts can find refuge in methadone maintenance clinics. About a thousand of them have been counted in methadone maintenance clinics around the country. Methadone maintenance is not a bad compromise for someone who has been addicted for 40 or 50 years. For such an individual the goal need not be eventual abstinence from all narcotics, as it would be for a younger person. Rather, one would consider keeping the elderly addict on methadone indefinitely if that is as far as he wants to go.

An alternative way to manage such a person is with periodic detoxifications to reduce the size of his habit because of the gradual buildup of tolerance. Although detoxification from narcotics is futile if abstinence is the goal, if we can accept a temporarily decreased opiate "habit" as a desirable end, then two or three detoxifications a year is not really a wasted effort.

Medical Addicts

The medical, or iatrogenic, addict is one who has become addicted while being treated for some painful illness, usually a malignancy that runs an unexpectedly benign course, but often enough for pancreatitis, arthritis, low back pain, or postsurgical pain. The management of chronic pain is one of the more difficult problems in medicine. Not every medical addict represents a medical error. Those who are going to die within a short time should be kept as comfortable as possible and given sufficient analgesics. When such a person happens to survive a year or years in pain, the addiction becomes a vexing problem for the patient, his family, and his physician. With considerable ingenuity and effort even these ill and hurting people can be detoxified and managed. Surely, highly addicting narcotics should not be prescribed for such recurrent, non-lethal conditions as migraine or asthma. There is good reason to believe that excellent analgesics will become available that have a lower dependency-producing potential than those now at hand.

Some medical addicts have been known to search out street heroin when legitimate supplies are denied them. Detoxification with methadone should occur in a hospital and proceed slowly. The stress of an abrupt withdrawal may be too much for a depleted, medically ill person.

Southern-type Addicts

A third category of elderly opiate addicts is represented by the individual who became overinvolved with paregoric, codeine cough syrups, or patent medicines containing opium during the days when these medicaments were easier to obtain than at present. Since that time they may have continued to receive some narcotic from a sympathetic doctor, especially if they happened to live in a small town. This is the so-called Southern type of addiction. It was not unusual at the turn of the century for a woman, less frequently a man, with chronic complaints to be maintained on morphine or Pantopon for years. It was predominantly a Southern rural phenomenon, but was by no means restricted to that area.

SEDATIVE AND TRANQUILIZER DEPENDENCE

Prescriptions for sleeping pills and minor tranquilizers are at an all-time high. Two of the most common complaints among elderly patients are insomnia and nervousness. These medications give initial relief, but as tolerance develops either more is needed or the effect wanes. When large amounts are consumed, mental confusion and physical clumsiness may develop. Old patients with a marginal mental compensation are easily pushed into a delirium. This is manifested by perplexity, an impaired ability to process information, memory and concentration disturbances, and a fluctuating loss of orientation, especially for time. Nor is sudden withdrawal of the medication likely to solve the problem. Indeed, it can be catastrophic with the oldster precipitated into the delirium tremens.

It is difficult to understand how one capsule of a sleeping medication every night can be effective over years, except as a conditioned stimulus. It has been found that insomniacs on constant doses of sleeping medication after a few months sleep no more than insomniacs not given any medication. In both instances sleep was broken, without deep sleep components (Stages III and IV), and sleep latency (falling asleep time) was prolonged. Nevertheless, both groups managed to obtain more than 5 hours of sleep during the night, the minimum requirement for people over 60.

Most sleeping pills suppress dreaming sleep. When they are discontinued or reduced, a dream time overshoot occurs resulting in vivid nightmares, which wake the sleeper. As indicated, the old person, even if he is well, has a reduced ability to detoxify ingested chemicals. Furthermore, his reduced capacity to compensate behaviorally for the drug intoxication makes him accident prone. The old person has little reserve with which to adjust to agents that alter his thinking and perception.

The repertoire of a physician's sleep procurement program need not have as its keystone the barbiturate and non-barbiturate sedatives. The bulk of complaints of geriatric insomnia are the result of either ignorance of what normal sleep patterns are in old folks, or they are due to secondary causes. In the first instance it is clear that the sleep requirement is reduced with aging, 4½ to 5½ hours being the physiologic need for those over 65. Another trick that the changing sleep pattern plays on the elderly is that Stages III and IV sleep, the deepest stages, are diminished or non-existent. Therefore, they may not have the feeling that they really slept. In addition, they may dream about being awake and claim the next day that they didn't close their eyes. All-night sleep tracings of such insomniacs indicate that although they did not fall asleep quickly, woke a number of times during the night, and were awake at an early hour, they still slept more than the minimum requirement.

Nocturnal pain, itching, muscle cramps, depression, and many other conditions can cause sleeplessness. For example, the need to void three or four times a night may be incompatible with proper sleep. It makes more sense to eliminate these sleep-disrupting factors than to mask them with hypnotics. Even when the insomnia seems to have no apparent cause that can be treated, there is no need to resort to sleeping potions immediately. Instead, a program of conditioning the patient should be planned that will encourage the onset of sleep. A pre-sleep ritual must be worked out and regularly followed. It would include hot drinks, warm baths, relaxation exercises, boring reading materials, and similar activities. If chemical therapy is needed, it should not be forgotten that certain antihistamines and minor tranquilizers like diazepam are as potent and effective as any hypnotic. By using these groups of agents along with the traditional sedatives in short one- or two-week courses, tolerances can be avoided. A part of the effectiveness of any sleeping pill is that it acts as a conditioning agent. Therefore, a placebo may be effective for some.

A person who tends to become dependent upon mind-altering chemicals should not be treated for his tension with drugs that have a record of being abused. Immature, rather inadequate, unstable persons with a poor tolerance for frustration are liable to become overinvolved in drugs that reduce anxiety, and distance the person from life stress, especially if the drugs happen to produce a measure of euphoria. Such an individual with a high anxiety level can be treated with small doses of the phenothiazines without risk of producing a dependency. Hydroxyzine is another drug that almost never causes habituation.

The senior citizen's nursing home problem requires separate mention. The oversedation of many nursing home members is a part of a general picture of overmedication. In part, this results from piling on drug orders without a periodic review of the chart to eliminate the unnecessary, but long-forgotten, items. Furthermore, eccentricity, non-conformity, even irascibility, are not indications for sedation. Our problem is that we have pills easily capable of making the crotchety compliant, the demanding dulled, and the surly sedated. Why should the busy staff put up with any disrupting influence whatsoever? One answer is that we don't want to obliterate chemically all personality features, however obstreperous. Another answer is that these drugs have side effects, which require other drugs, which have side effects.

Since the source of geriatric sedative abuse is, almost invariably, the physician's order or prescription, more enlightened prescribing practices could do a good deal to solve the problem. Large quantities of sedatives should not be available to confused, elderly patients. They will inevitably be misused. When such patients escalate their intake to the equivalent of eight 100 mg secobarbital capsules in 24 hours, hospitalization is necessary for slow detoxification, support of cardiovascular function, and the prevention of convulsions.

PROPRIETARY MEDICINE ABUSE

There is a wide range of patent medicines that can be abused by the aged. The over-the-counter sleeping potions contain an antihistamine with or without a small amount of scopolamine. The wake-up pills are usually caffeine or an ephedrine-like compound. An enormous market for analgesics exists, and aspirin, an aspirin-phenacetin-caffeine combination, or other salicylates, are widely used. These preparations can be incorrectly used, for example, to take aspirin a number of times a day to prevent headache. None of these drugs are innocuous—certainly not aspirin, and toxic effects are not rare.

Despite all the warnings about bromides, their use as tranquilizers and analgesics persists. Four patent medicines containing one or more bromide salts are available: Bromo Seltzer, Alva Tranquil, Miles Nervine, and Lanabrom Elixer. Another, Neurosine, requires a doctor's prescription. The typical person who becomes overinvolved in chronic bromide intoxication is a white female over 40. Bromism and alcoholism are often associated. A blood bromide level of over 80 mg percent ordinarily signifies that the mental confusion is bromide-related. However, a bromism is rarely considered in the differential diagnosis of delirium, and its role remains unrecognized. This is particularly true of those with cerebral arteriosclerosis, and they seem predisposed to develop a bromide psychosis.

GERIATRIC ALCOHOLISM

The most serious of all drug abuse problems involving the aged is alcoholism. Of 534 consecutive over-60 patients admitted for psychiatric observation to San Francisco General Hospital, 28 percent had a serious drinking problem. Of these, 80 percent required hospitalization for their excessive drinking. A study reported from the medical service of the Harlem Hospital Center revealed that 63 percent of the men and 35 percent of the women were alcoholics. In a large house-to-house survey in the Washington Heights section of upper Manhattan, the peak incidence of alcohol abuse was found in the 45- to 54-year-old group. It was 2.3 percent in the 55- to 74-year-old group. If these figures can be extrapolated nationwide, it would mean that about a million people over the age of 55 are alcoholics.

Geriatric alcoholics can be readily subdivided into two groups. Those in the first group have had a lifelong history of excessive and destructive drinking practices, and have managed to avoid the lethal illnesses and injuries associated with such an existence. They are the last survivors of a much larger cohort of alcoholics. The outlook for abstinence is not good, although a small number do manage to stop drinking, with or without treatment. The second group consists of those who have started drinking heavily late in life. Not infrequently this has been in response to one or more of the losses that accompany aging: losses of loved ones, loss of self-esteem, and loss of feelings of worth. For their separation anxieties and situational depressions they have come to use alcohol as a form of self-treatment. It acts as a depressant, blocking the painful input from memory and from the environment. The prognosis is more favorable for this group. New interpersonal relationships must be formed, perhaps in a resocialization program. Sometimes, antidepressant medication is needed for a while. But it is usually the formation of a close relationship with one or a few people that changes their attitudes and saves them from a life that is bottled in bondage.

INDEX